CURRENT ORAL AND MAXILLOFACIAL IMAGING

CURRENT ORAL AND MAXILLOFACIAL IMAGING

Thomas F. Razmus, D.D.S., M.S.
Associate Professor
Department of Diagnostic Services
West Virginia University
School of Dentistry
Morgantown, West Virginia

Gail F. Williamson, R.D.H., M.S.
Associate Professor
Department of Oral Surgery, Medicine and Pathology
Indiana University
School of Dentistry
Indianapolis, Indiana

W.B. SAUNDERS COMPANY
A Division of Harcourt Brace & Company
Philadelphia   London   Toronto   Montreal   Sydney   Tokyo

W.B. SAUNDERS COMPANY
A Division of Harcourt Brace & Company

The Curtis Center
Independence Square West
Philadelphia, Pennsylvania 19106

Library of Congress Cataloging-in-Publication Data

Current oral and maxillofacial imaging / Thomas F. Razmus, Gail F. Williamson.—
1st ed.

    p. cm.

ISBN 0–7216–4005–2

1. Teeth—Imaging.   2. Jaws—Imaging.   3. Mouth—
    Imaging. I. Williamson, Gail F. II. Title. [DNLM: 1. Radiography,
    Dental—methods.   2. Diagnostic Imaging—methods.   3. Stomatognathic
    System—radiography.   WN 230 R278c 1996]

RK308.5.R39   1996   617.5′20754—dc20

DNLM/DLC   95-37883

Current Oral and Maxillofacial Imaging   ISBN 0–7216–4005–2

Printed in the United States of America

Last digit is the print number: 9   8   7   6   5   4   3   2   1

PREFACE

Dentistry, in the past decade, has been introduced to new levels of sophistication in diagnostic technology. Advances in imaging the structures in and around the oral cavity have evolved in concert with associated computer hardware and software. New ways to image the oral and maxillofacial complex require new knowledge and skills, as well as a firm understanding of the basic principles of conventional radiology. The authors have attempted to intertwine the basic principles of film-based (conventional) radiology with those of state-of-the-art computer-assisted imaging throughout this textbook.

Chapter 1, "An Overview of Oral and Maxillofacial Imaging," provides the reader with the mechanism of image formation and applications of the various methods used to image the teeth, adjacent bone, and surrounding structures in the oral and maxillofacial region.

In Chapter 2, "X Rays—Their Source and Behavior," atomic structure related to the production of x rays in the diagnostic energy range is discussed. The basic principles of x-ray production by an x-ray machine are presented. Because images produced by both film-based and electronic or computer-assisted systems require x rays to carry patient information to the image receptor, an understanding of the behavior of x rays is essential. In addition, the safe and efficient use of x rays requires that x-ray generating equipment be in optimum working condition. Quality assurance tests provide the means of assessing the operating status of such equipment.

"Characteristics of Image Receptors and Producing Diagnostic Quality Images," Chapter 3, presents a discussion of image receptors including direct exposure film, light-sensitive film and intensifying screen systems, and charge-coupled devices or electronic image receptors. Although x rays are the common denominator among these imaging methods, the mechanism by which each system creates an image is quite different. The principles of each system are discussed and similarities and differences are pointed out.

Chapter 4, "The Biological Effects and Safe Use of Radiation," addresses ionizing and nonionizing forms of radiation applied to diagnostic imaging tasks. Radiation safety and dose reduction practices are discussed in light of the risk of incurring harmful biological effects. The principles of x-ray behavior and radiation safety are applied to the design of a radiation-safe dental facility. The practice of radiology requires the use of various environmentally harmful materials. A discussion of the proper handling and disposal of these materials is included.

"Intraoral Radiographic Techniques," Chapter 5, introduces the reader to various intraoral film types, intraoral electronic image receptors, and techniques employed to obtain high-quality images. Images that demonstrate the result of the more commonly committed technical errors are presented. At times, anatomic variation or other patient-related variables make it difficult to apply the principles of optimal image production: a discussion of difficult image receptor placement situations is included.

Chapter 6, "Radiographic Infection Control," focuses on the prevention of contamination in the dental environment of the operator, x-ray machine, and darkroom equipment by the patient's oral fluids. Environmental protective barriers are utilized to prevent primary exposure of the operator and environmental surfaces to contaminants. A variety of protocols exist to transport saliva- or blood-contaminated film from the operatory to the processor. Inadvertent contamination at some point in the treatment sequence is likely to occur, so clean-up procedures must be standardized and practiced consistently.

Application of the principles presented in Chapter 7, "Darkroom Film Processing and Quality Assurance," will help ensure the production of consistently high quality images with minimal exposure and expense. An image obtained using perfect technique can be rendered useless through improper handling of the film or problems with the processing system. Darkroom quality assurance procedures are designed to monitor performance of the processing chemicals and the processor.

The dentist can perform a comprehensive assessment of the oral and maxillofacial structures by utilizing "Panoramic Radiography, Other Extraoral Projections, and Implant Site Assessment," Chapter 8. Although image receptor placement relative to the patient is critical in all imaging methods, the diagnostic quality of a panoramic image is highly dependent on properly positioning a patient in the panoramic machine. The panoramic projection is the most common extraoral view, and clinicians must be able to evaluate the anatomic accuracy of the image before making diagnostic judgments. The assessment of potential sites for implant placement requires adequate visualization in the mesial-distal, superior-inferior, and buccal-lingual dimensions. Several methods of obtaining this information exist.

Chapter 9, "Radiographic Interpretation—Describing What You See," is the culmination of producing a diagnostic quality image. A dental professional responsible for producing diagnostic images should also possess the ability to describe the features of the resultant image. Description of radiographic features using standardized terminology in a consistent manner is essential for meaningful communication. This chapter does not include the names of radiographic lesions but does present the essentials of proper viewing conditions, a limited vocabulary of commonly used radiographic descriptive terminology, and several images and legends that illustrate the application of this terminology.

We hope that dental students, allied dental health students, and the practicing dental team will find this text to be a useful reference for state-of-the-art technical information and a resource for problem-solving in daily practice.

THOMAS F. RAZMUS
GAIL F. WILLIAMSON

ACKNOWLEDGMENTS

The authors would like to express their appreciation to the Dr. Norman H. Baker Endowment Fund, West Virginia University Foundation, Inc., for the partial funding of art and photography.

Individuals deserving special thanks are Dr. Myron Kasle, for providing us with the opportunity to write this textbook; Ms. Debra Kirby, for her hours spent editing the drafts of the manuscript; Mr. Paul A. Dombrowski and Ms. Dawn W. Dombrowski, biomedical photographers, and Ms. Carol Grimes, Senior Biomedical Designer, in the Department of Biomedical Communications at West Virginia University Health Sciences Center; and Mr. Mark A. Dirlam, graphic artist, Mr. Mike Halloran, photographer, and Mrs. Alana L. Barra, Supervisor, in the Department of Illustrations at Indiana University School of Dentistry.

Special thanks to the following West Virginia University School of Dentistry and Indiana University School of Dentistry students for taking time from their already busy schedules to "model" for several of the technical photographs: Mr. Gerald Clark, Ms. Merin Kunukkasseril, Ms. Zahra Loynab, Mr. Rory McClaurin, Mr. Troy McGrew, Ms. Roxane Oshiro, Mr. Michael Perez, and Mr. Khoi H. Vu, as well as Indiana University School of Dentistry staff member Mrs. Heather Hoffmeyer, CDA.

The following individuals contributed valuable and very much appreciated illustrative materials: Dr. Cecil E. Brown, Jr., Indianapolis, Indiana; Dr. Brent Dove, San Antonio, Texas; Dr. Jerry Katz, Kansas City, Missouri; Dr. Curt Lundeen, Portland, Oregon; Dr. Ted Parks, Indianapolis, Indiana; and Dr. Jerry Pifer, Morgantown, West Virginia. We thank you all.

THOMAS F. RAZMUS
GAIL F. WILLIAMSON

CONTENTS

1

AN OVERVIEW OF ORAL AND MAXILLOFACIAL IMAGING

THOMAS F. RAZMUS

In 1895, Wilhelm Konrad Roentgen discovered, quite by accident, the mysterious energy that he called the *x ray*. Over the ensuing 100 years, we have learned about the nature of x-ray energy, how to generate it, and how to manipulate it to accomplish different tasks. The health sciences, industry, and ultimately the public have been the beneficiaries of Roentgen's discovery. We have also come to learn of the damage x-ray energy can cause to living systems. Historically, the inadvertent exposure of certain populations to high doses of x radiation during peace and wartime has resulted in sources of research data. Radiation safety principles and guidelines have been developed from the data collected on these populations.

The last century has seen the development of increasingly sophisticated x-ray imaging equipment and modalities for use in dentistry and medicine. Research and development in imaging with other forms of energy, such as radio frequency emissions (magnetic resonance), sound (ultrasound), heat (thermography), and internal source radiation (scintigraphy), has expanded our imaging flexibility and capabilities. Dentistry, particularly in the last decade, has begun to utilize imaging methods beyond the conventional x-ray machine, and this trend will continue. The term *dental radiology* is no longer adequate when speaking of imaging the oral and maxillofacial region.

INTRODUCTION

A photograph is the image of an object resulting from the interaction of *light rays,* the object, and the photographic film. The process of creating a photograph is known as *photography.* Analogous to photography is *radiography,* which uses *x rays* rather than light rays to produce an image. The interaction of the x rays passing through the object creates an image on the x-ray film called a *radiograph.* The study of the radiographic process and the information presented by radiographs is the science of *radiology.*

Sophisticated diagnostic imaging methods that originated in medicine have been adapted for use in the oral and maxillofacial region and are available to the contemporary dentist and allied dental professional. This chapter updates and educates the practitioner in the spectrum of modalities available to create diagnostic images of the head and neck.

INTRAORAL RADIOGRAPHY

Intraoral radiography is the standard technique for obtaining diagnostic information concerning structures in and about the mouth, primarily the teeth (dentition) and alveolar bone. The x-ray machine used in this technique can be seen in most dental offices and is referred to as an intraoral x-ray machine.

An *intraoral radiograph* results when an x-ray film packet is placed in the mouth and the x-ray beam is directed in such a way that it passes through the objects of interest and interacts with the film to create an image. There are three types of intraoral radiographs: periapical, bitewing, and occlusal. Each film type has a primary purpose, i.e., a periapical and a bitewing radiograph of the same area will each present slightly different information (Fig. 1–1). Intraoral radiographic techniques are discussed in Chapter 5.

EXTRAORAL RADIOGRAPHY

Extraoral radiographs are made with the radiographic film located outside the patient. The film and x-ray source are positioned on opposite sides of the patient's head. The x-ray beam is directed at the area of interest in such a way that the object's image is projected onto the film. Most extraoral radiographs are made using a standard intraoral x-ray machine in a dental operatory, an extraoral x-ray machine such as a cephalometric unit common to an orthodontist's office, or a medical x-ray unit as found in a hospital.

Certain types of extraoral radiographs require motion of the x-ray source and the film to create an image. These techniques are referred to as *tomography,* or cross-sectional radiography, and require specialized machines. The

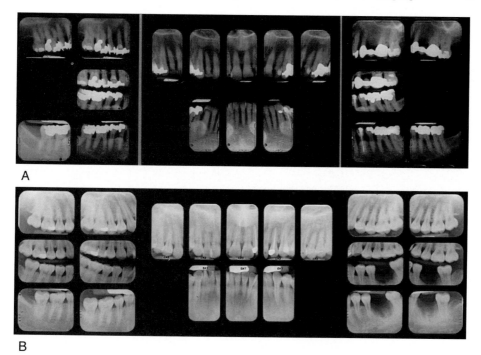

Figure 1–1. Typical full-mouth surveys of intraoral radiographs. Periapical radiographs are those that demonstrate the entire length of the roots of the teeth and the bone surrounding the roots. Bitewing radiographs are those that portray the crowns of the teeth and the alveolar crest bone adjacent to the teeth. *A,* This survey exhibits greater overall density and contrast than the survey in *B.*

result of the motion of the film and x-ray source is to depict on the film a predetermined layer of structures from within the patient. This layer can range in thickness from 2 to 4 mm or more. Objects outside this layer are blurred and will minimally obscure the objects of interest within the sharply depicted layer.

There are two types of tomography: *conventional* tomography in which the film and x-ray source move parallel to one another with the patient in between, and *rotational* tomography in which the film and x-ray source move around the patient in a circular path. Rotational tomography is generally known as *panoramic radiography* (Fig. 1–2).

Conventional tomography is task-oriented. The clinician is seeking specific information when making and viewing a tomograph. Most tomographic machines create an image in the sagittal and coronal (frontal) planes and at angular degrees between these planes (Fig. 1–3). The most common tomographic "slice of information" is 2 mm thick, although slice thickness can be varied. Tomographic images are most commonly used to examine specific predetermined sections of the paranasal sinuses, temporomandibular joints, and potential implant placement sites. Techniques can be designed to image most any region of the oral and maxillofacial complex. Conventional tomography will produce an image that represents a flat plane through the patient, whereas a panoramic image will represent a generally horseshoe-shaped

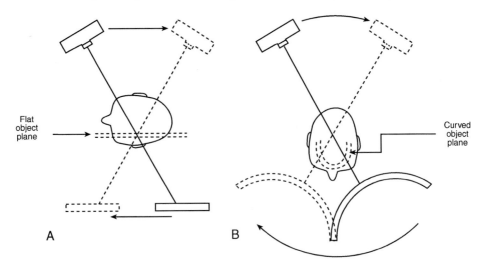

Figure 1–2. Tomographic object planes. Conventional tomography (*A*) creates an image of a flat object plane, whereas rotational tomography (*B*) results in an image of a curved object plane from within the patient.

plane from within the patient. The panoramic image slice corresponds closely to the arch form of the teeth and alveolar bone.

The most common extraoral radiograph is the *panoramic* radiograph made with a panoramic x-ray machine. These are highly specialized machines that are extremely sensitive to technique errors. Images are produced when the film and x-ray source rotate around a precisely positioned patient. Inattention to how the patient is placed in the machine will result in distortion of the resultant image that may compromise diagnostic accuracy. A panoramic image must be evaluated for technique errors and artifacts prior to attempting to obtain diagnostic information from the radiograph. Errors in technique, particularly in how the patient is positioned in the machine, will produce characteristic distortions in the resultant images. The clinician must be capable of recognizing these distortions, correlating the findings with the appropriate error, and making a decision regarding the diagnostic quality of the image before attempting to gain information about the patient from the radiograph.

Panoramic radiographs provide broad anatomical coverage, as the name implies. The image consists of a spread-out and flattened representation of the patient's skull (Fig. 1–4). Most panoramic images will portray the lower half of the orbits superiorly to just below the chin inferiorly, and they will extend bilaterally to include the condyles. The experienced clinician will be able to visualize a skull when observing a panoramic image. A technique that might help the novice become oriented to the panoramic image is to view the film with the letter "L" (patient's left side) in the lower right corner, then curve the film back as if wrapping it around a large coffee can and begin to visualize and trace the major anatomical structures: orbit, malar process, zygomatic arch, articular eminence, condyle, and so on. This study aid becomes especially valuable if a skull is substituted for the coffee can.

Panoramic radiographs provide a means for the general assessment of the

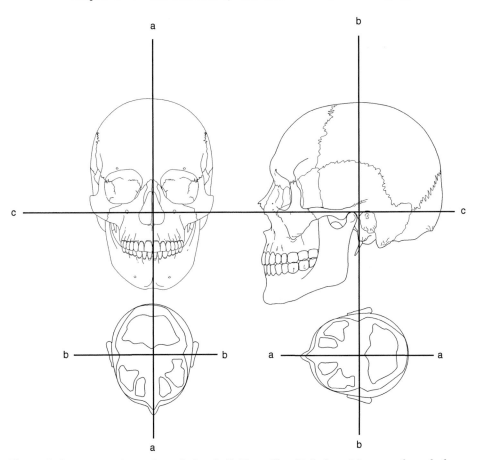

Figure 1–3. Imaging planes through the skull. The midsagittal plane (*a*) passes through the center of the skull from anterior to posterior, divides the skull into right and left halves, and is perpendicular to the floor and the frontal or coronal plane. When not located at the midline of the skull, it is simply referred to as a sagittal plane. The coronal or frontal plane (*b*) divides the skull into anterior and posterior segments and will be at right angles to any sagittal plane. The axial plane (*c*) lies at right angles to the long axis of the body and to any sagittal or frontal (coronal) plane. The lower pair of diagrams represent anatomical structures sectioned through the axial plane at *c*.

region portrayed. Panoramic images are useful for detecting large carious lesions and associated apical pathosis, severe periodontal bone loss, large deposits of calculus, previously undetected impacted teeth, and jaw fractures. A general assessment can be made concerning potential implant sites, alveolar bone height, morphology of the condyles, gross irregularities of the maxillary sinuses, structures located near to but outside the mandible, and generalized changes in the trabecular pattern of the maxilla and mandible associated with systemic disease. Carefully made serial panoramic radiographs can be useful to assess growth and development.

Although the manufacturers of panoramic machines are constantly improving the quality of the images produced by their respective machines, clinicians should not depend on these images for high-resolution tasks. In dentistry, the panoramic technique does not replace conventional radiography, but, when used as a supplemental diagnostic procedure, it does result in a compre-

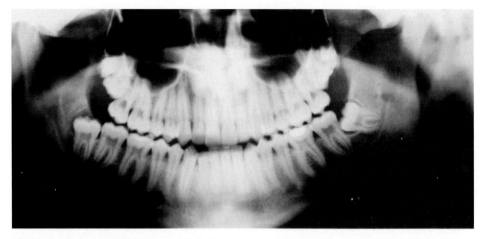

Figure 1–4. A panoramic image of high diagnostic quality. Note the gentle upward curve of the occlusal plane (the "smile line"); the symmetry of width between the rami, and the molars and premolars bilaterally; the well-defined images of the anterior teeth, and the roots of the maxillary molars and premolars; and the minimal overlapping of interproximal contacts.

hensive radiographic survey more complete than the intraoral series alone. Panoramic radiography and other extraoral projections are discussed in Chapter 8.

ELECTRONIC IMAGING

Electronic imaging is not a new concept. The most common device is the television set. Other forms of common electronic imaging include the real-time image seen in the viewing screen of a camcorder, or the display on a computer screen. Medicine has been producing electronic images with diagnostic x rays for many years; dentistry has just begun to apply this technology to the oral and maxillofacial region. In the last 10 years or so, there has been a tremendous increase in computer-based imaging technology in dentistry. Ensuing discussions will address the use of electronic intraoral image receptors, methods of digital image acquisition, image enhancement, and computer-aided image analysis.

Recall that light reacts with photographic film to create a photograph, and x rays interact with x-ray film to make a radiograph. These imaging modalities are referred to as *film-based imaging*. The light or x-ray energy interacts with the electrons in the chemical emulsion of the film (image receptor) in film-based imaging. A film-based image is recorded on the film as an invisible (latent) image until processed in the darkroom. An electronic image also results from an electron interaction but is processed by a computer. The image receptor in this case is an electronic detector or sensor.

Film-based images or radiographs are *analog* images. The electronic image seen on a computer screen is a *digital* image. Use of the term "digital" simply means that a computer has processed the image. Generally speaking, an analog image is characterized by continuous gradations from one area of the image to the next. An analog image, whether a radiograph or a color photograph, exhibits gradual changes from one color or shade to another. The human eye may not be capable of distinguishing an analog image from a digital image, depending on the degree of computer processing to which the digital image has been subjected.

A digital image results from the conversion of analog data to digital data (Fig. 1–5). To accomplish this, analog data are quantified or assigned numerical values. Wrist watches comprise a group of common analog and digital devices that quantify increments of time in different ways. A wrist watch with traditional hands is an analog device; a watch that displays the time as a discrete number is a digital device. You might say that a digital clock readout is more exact when compared with the constantly moving hands of an analog timepiece. Digital information is contained in, and presented as, discrete units of information. In digital electronic images, these discrete units of information are referred to as *pixels,* or "picture elements" (Fig. 1–6).

Two methods that result in an image that has been processed by a computer are (1) digitized film radiography, and (2) direct digital radiography. *Digitized film radiography* starts with a conventional radiograph, a film-based analog image, that is converted to a digital image (Fig. 1–7). *Direct digital radiography (imaging),* often referred to as "filmless radiography," uses an electronic sensor in place of the film. The terms "digital" or "digitized" indicate that the images will be generated by a computer, and thus will be able to be manipulated.

A film-based image, such as a conventional radiograph, is made up of continuous shades (analog data) of gray between the extremes of black and white. Each shade of gray possesses a certain *optical density,* which is related to the amount of light that can pass through the image at that particular site. Computers cannot display an image of analog data. An *analog-to-digital converter,* or "frame grabber," is used to digitize or convert the analog (contin-

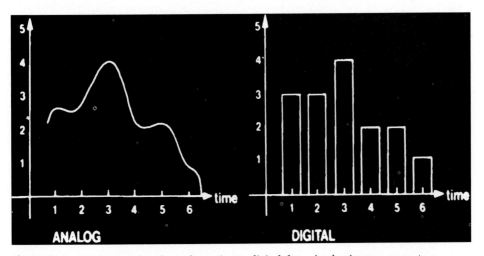

Figure 1–5. Conversion of analog information to digital data. Analog images present as gradual and continuous changes from one intensity or shade of gray to another. Digital conversion transforms the nondiscrete variations in analog image intensity into discrete and quantifiable units of change in intensity. Each unit of change in intensity in a digital image is represented by a pixel, or "picture element." (Courtesy of Dr. S. Brent Dove, University of Texas Dental School at San Antonio, Texas.)

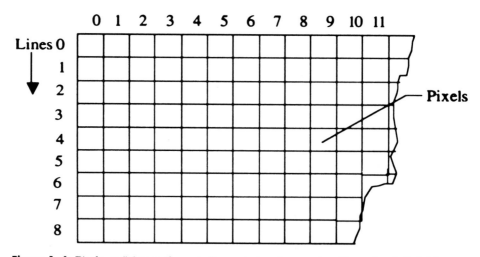

Figure 1-6. Pixels, or "picture elements," are what make up a two-dimensional digital image. Each square, or pixel, is assigned a number that corresponds to the analog gray scale intensity that it represents in the digital image. The size and number of pixels in a given area contribute to digital image quality. (Courtesy of Dr. S. Brent Dove, University of Texas Dental School at San Antonio, Texas.)

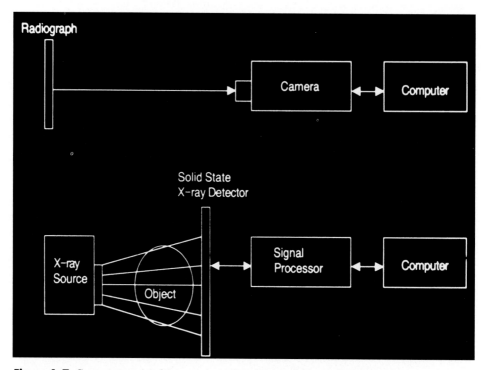

Figure 1-7. Computer-assisted image processing. Digitized film radiography starts with a conventional radiograph. A video camera scans the radiographic image and transfers the information to a computer for processing. Direct digital radiography employs a CCD, an electronic solid state x-ray detector or sensor in place of film to obtain the initial image. Electronic signals from the sensor transfer image data to a computer. (Courtesy of Dr. S. Brent Dove, University of Texas Dental School at San Antonio, Texas.)

uous scale) information into digital (discrete units) information. The digitization of a conventional radiographic image involves conversion of the continuous scale of grays into a pattern (an array) of squares (pixels). Each pixel is given a number value that corresponds to a certain gray shade or optical density. This results in the film image being transformed into a two-dimensional array of numbers, termed picture elements or pixels. A computer is able to store the information in this numeric format. In summary, digitized film radiography involves placement of a radiograph on a viewbox and scanning of the backlit image with a video camera or similar light-sensitive device. An analog-to-digital converter then quantifies (digitizes) the analog signal transmitted from the light detector into digital data, which is stored in a computer (Fig. 1–8).

Direct digital image processing is the means by which electronic images are generated without film. This process allows acquisition, manipulation, and immediate display of a patient's images. In electronic image production, the film (*image receptor*) is replaced by a type of electronic image receptor called a *charge-coupled device* (CCD). The invisible image captured by the CCD is electronically transferred to an image processor and then to a computer monitor for immediate viewing (see Fig. 1–7).

The electronic image, whether digitized from film or acquired directly, can be manipulated (adjusted) while being viewed (Fig. 1–9). Various presentations of the image can be printed or saved in the computer's memory for later study. Electronic images can be transferred by telecommunication technology to other locations for viewing and study by several people at the same time. A conventional film-based image, on the other hand, cannot be manipulated, must be stored as a piece of film, and must be physically sent to other locations as the original or as a duplicate film.

Equipment for *"filmless"* or *intraoral direct digital radiography* is available from several commercial sources. Although the list of manufacturers is constantly growing and the technology continues to improve, available systems use slightly different methods to capture and process an image. Standardization among manufacturers would allow facilities with different brands of equipment to transfer information among themselves more easily.

SUBTRACTION AND DIGITAL SUBTRACTION RADIOGRAPHY

The subtraction technique is useful to detect subtle differences between radiographs made of the same structure(s) at different times. *Subtraction radiography* allows the clinician to see subtle changes that have occurred over time more clearly. This is accomplished by removing or *subtracting* from the two images all the information that is unchanged. The result is a third image, the *subtracted image,* that portrays only the differences between the first two images. Structures that have not changed detract from the quality of the image and are referred to as *structured noise.* Subtraction radiography removes all anatomical structures that have not changed (structured noise) between subsequent radiographic examinations, thus allowing the clinician to more easily see changes in diagnostically significant information. Elimination of the structured noise results in an image that clearly depicts only the changes on a gray background (Fig. 1–10).

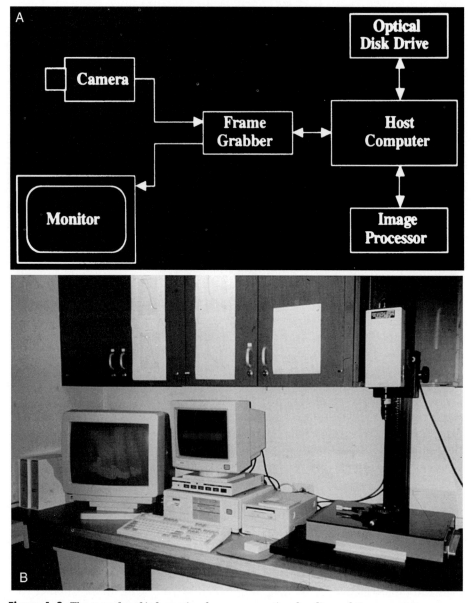

Figure 1–8. The transfer of information from a conventional radiograph to a computer requires specialized equipment. A "framegrabber" converts the analog data to a digital format so the computer can understand it. Once processed by the computer, the image can be viewed and manipulated on the monitor. *A,* A schematic of this process. *B,* An analog-to-digital imaging workstation. The video camera is on the right, and two monitors and a computer are to the left. (Courtesy of Dr. S. Brent Dove, University of Texas Dental School at San Antonio, Texas.)

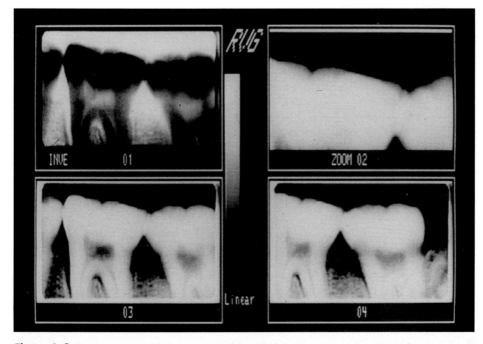

Figure 1–9. Images on a computer screen. Although these images were generated using an intraoral electronic x-ray detector or image receptor, their appearance on a monitor would be similar to that of digitized conventional radiographic images. Note how the features of the image can be manipulated. (Courtesy of Dr. S. Brent Dove, University of Texas Dental School at San Antonio, Texas.)

Application of the subtraction technique has certain requirements. The two images made at different times must be as identical as possible. The exposure factors and processing parameters that affect density and contrast must be consistent between the two radiographs, and the projection geometry must be duplicated as nearly as possible. Prior to the application of digital imaging technology, subtraction radiography was not practical for intraoral applications.

Historically, subtraction radiography developed as a technique that used radiographic film, photographic techniques to create positive and negative images, a viewbox, and the human eye to align and superimpose the images to be subtracted. Each of these steps introduced errors into a method of imaging that depended upon standardization to produce an optimal result.

The introduction of the computer to image processing has eliminated most of the cumulative effects of these errors by correcting for them. Computers use special programs called *algorithms* to make these adjustments. Computer algorithms are meant to compensate for minor variations in density, contrast, and projection geometry. Even with computerized image processing, subtraction radiography requires strict control of exposure factors, processing parameters, and projection geometry. Subtraction can be performed on images that have been digitized from radiographs or on images acquired through direct digital imaging.

Digital subtraction radiography is useful in dentistry to assess changes

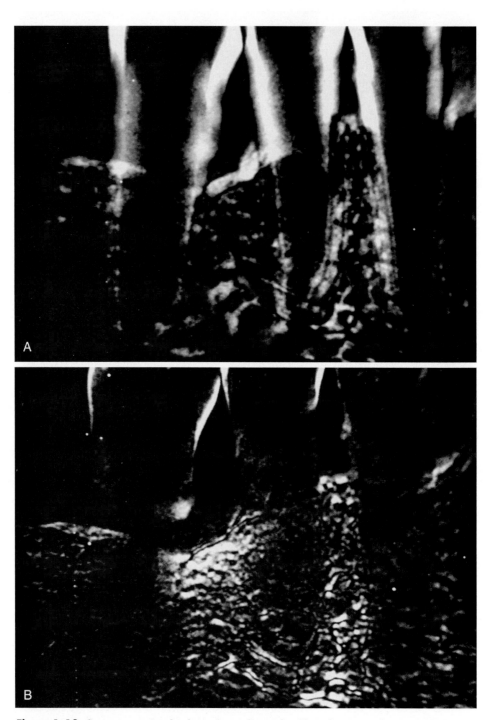

Figure 1-10. Computer-assisted subtraction radiography. Note the reversed contrast in *A, B,* and *C* in which the normally dark and light areas of the image are reversed. *A,* Initial radiograph demonstrating interproximal crestal bone. *B,* Subsequent image demonstrating changes of interproximal bone.

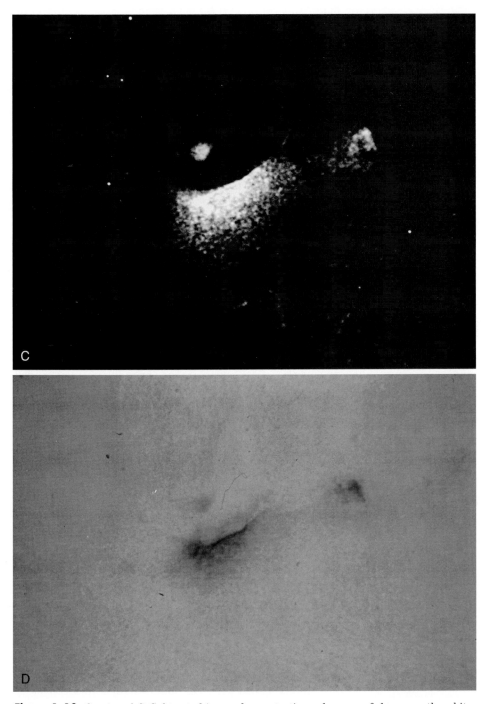

Figure 1-10. *Continued C,* Subtracted image demonstrating only areas of change as the white regions. *D,* Subtracted image with normal contrast scale that demonstrates areas of change as the dark regions. (Courtesy of Dr. S. Brent Dove, University of Texas Dental School at San Antonio, Texas.)

over time in alveolar bone, the resolution or progression of periapical bone lesions, and the progression of caries.

COMPUTED TOMOGRAPHY

Computed tomography (CT) incorporates the principles of direct digital (computed) electronic imaging and cross-sectional radiography (tomography). The image in CT is produced by an x-ray source and electronic detectors that are positioned opposite each other and move synchronously around the long axis of the patient. As the synchronized movement progresses around the patient, attenuation data corresponding to a scan of 360° are transferred to a computer.

Recall that conventional or film-based tomography gives the viewer a relatively clear image of a preselected layer of anatomy by blurring the structures in front of and in back of the structures of interest. Conventional tomography of the head depends upon standard frontal (coronal) and lateral (sagittal) cross-sectional projections. Axial cross-sectional images of the head are difficult or impossible to obtain using x-ray film and an x-ray machine of any kind. The film-based projection that most closely approximates an axial cross-sectional view of the head is the submentovertex (SMV) or basilar projection. This projection requires that the film be placed on top of the patient's head and the beam directed through the chin. Most patients cannot extend their necks enough to allow the beam to project an image through the long axis of the skull. Computed tomography, on the other hand, creates axial cross-sectional images routinely. Refer to Figure 1–3 for a review of the imaging planes through the skull.

The standard CT image is made in the axial plane. The patient is positioned horizontally in a CT machine, and the x-ray detectors are arranged axially around the patient. The x-ray beam is directed perpendicular to the long axis of the patient's body and passes through the patient to reach the detectors. Slices in the axial plane will be perpendicular to the long axis of the patient's body, unless the position of the patient is changed within the gantry or the gantry is tilted. The gantry is a doughnut-shaped device in which are located the x-ray source and detectors and into which the patient is placed. The detectors transfer information about a complete slice through the region of interest to the computer. Slices may range in thickness from 1.5 to 10.0 mm, depending on the anatomical site. The computer capability allows several axial images to be made in sequence through the entire region of interest. Each layer may be studied separately or in sequence to follow the anatomical extension of the findings.

Advantages of CT include its ability to reformat a sequence of axial images into images of other planes (Fig. 1–11) or into three-dimensional images (Fig. 1–12). Computed tomographic imaging can also depict subtle differences in tissue densities much more effectively than can film-based radiographic techniques. Intravenous contrast media can be used to differentiate one soft tissue type from another even further.

The CT image is, generally speaking, a direct digital image consisting of pixels (picture elements), as mentioned in earlier discussions. A major difference between CT and digitized film radiography, and between CT and direct

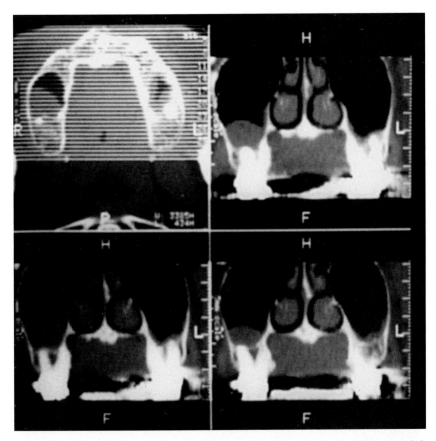

Figure 1-11. Axial and reformatted coronal computed tomography images. The upper left image is the axial image from which the various coronal images have been constructed. The horizontal lines across the axial image correspond to specific coronal planes that can be constructed and viewed. (Courtesy of Dr. S. Brent Dove, University of Texas Dental School at San Antonio, Texas.)

digital imaging, is that the *CT image pixels* represent a three-dimensional volume element, called a *voxel*. The image seen on the computer monitor of a CT console possesses the additional dimension of depth.

CT is especially useful when a pathological process is suspected of having extended beyond the limits of bone into surrounding soft tissues. Lesions limited to the bones of the maxilla or mandible can be studied with intraoral or extraoral film-based imaging.

In most cases, mandibular fractures are easy to visualize on panoramic and other extraoral projections. Assessment of the extent of fractures of the maxillofacial structures may be inadequate if only film-based images are used. When the complex bones of the face and skull are involved, the unobstructed views provided by the thin serial slices of CT are essential to help determine the true extent of bone damage.

Thin serial CT slices (1.5 mm) can be reformatted by computer to present a three-dimensional image of the region of interest. The three-dimensional image can be rotated on the computer screen. Computer software exists that can add color to selected structures and can even allow removal of all parts

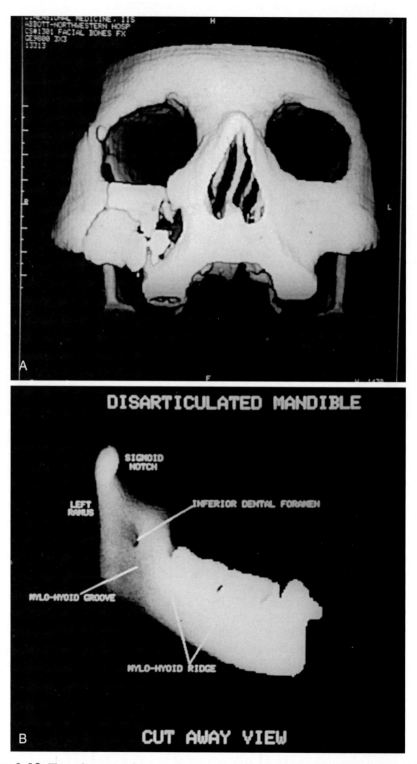

Figure 1-12. Three-dimensional images from computed tomography (CT) data. *A,* Selected portion of a skull constructed from CT data to help analyze the fracture of facial bones on the right side. *B,* Portion of a mandible constructed from CT data to demonstrate normal anatomy. (Courtesy of Dr. S. Brent Dove, University of Texas Dental School at San Antonio, Texas.)

of the image not involved with the structure of interest, a process called *disarticulation* (Fig. 1–12*B*). Since all the data collected while the patient is being imaged are stored in the computer, the patient need not be present for manipulation of the image.

Imaging the temporomandibular joints (TMJ) with CT has evolved into a task-oriented diagnostic tool. Initially, investigators were confident that CT would be the modality of choice to image the TMJ. As research progressed, it was found that the articular disk, a cartilaginous structure, was not imaged as well as had been anticipated. Images of the articular disk are only moderately well defined, whereas bony anatomy produces very high resolution pictures. Computed tomography has remained the technique of choice for evaluating bony changes affecting the condyle and articular eminence in patients who have received certain types of TMJ implants. Clinical findings and the results of a film-based examination suggesting perforation of the glenoid fossa and involvement of the middle cranial fossa should prompt the clinician to order a CT examination.

Perhaps the most exciting application of CT in dentistry is the assessment of patients for dental implant placement (Fig. 1–13). Computer software dedicated to this application provides a CT image designed specifically for preoperative assessment of the maxilla and mandible for placement of osseointegrated implants. Still other software packages can generate a model of a mandible from reformatted data upon which a subperiosteal implant framework can be fabricated. This may be familiar to you as "computer-aided design/computer-aided manufacturing" or "CAD/CAM." Several film-based and CT imaging applications, including implant site assessment, are presented in Chapter 8.

MAGNETIC RESONANCE IMAGING

Magnetic resonance imaging (MRI) does not use x rays (ionizing radiation) to form its diagnostic image. MRI depends upon the *hydrogen atoms* in the body reacting in a certain way in a *magnetic field*. Why hydrogen atoms? Because our bodies are made primarily of water, which contains an abundance of hydrogen atoms. Hydrogen atomic nuclei are especially susceptible to the force of an external magnetic field. What is the relationship of hydrogen atoms to magnetic fields and the formation of MR images? This explanation will involve some discussion of atomic nuclei, specifically of the hydrogen atom.

The nucleus of a hydrogen atom contains one proton and one neutron. A *proton* is a subatomic particle that possesses a *positive electric charge* and a motion called *spin*. Neutrons are electrically neutral and have their own spin. You could think of a hydrogen nucleus as a positively charged spinning "top." Another physical phenomenon is that a moving electric charge will produce a magnetic field. Thus, this electrically charged spinning top generates a magnetic field about itself that will have a north and south pole just like any magnet. The hydrogen nuclei in our bodies are essentially positively charged spinning tops, or tiny magnets. If one of these spinning tops were put on a table, it would spin on its south pole with the north pole at the other end of the axis of rotation and pointing generally upward. If several of these spin-

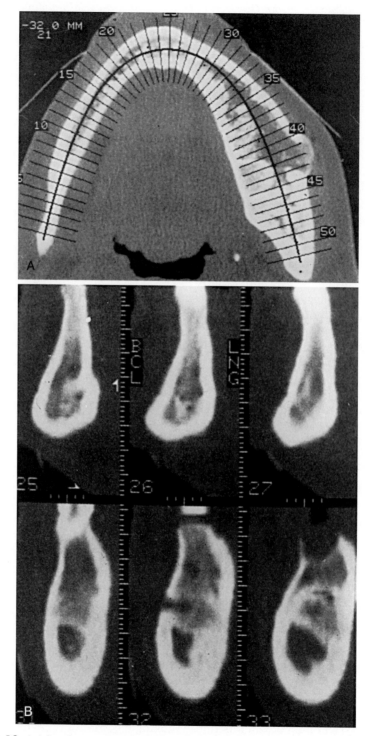

Figure 1-13. Axial and cross-sectional images of a mandible for implant site assessment. *A,* Axial image of the mandible. The inscribed arc generally corresponds to the buccal-lingual center of the bone being imaged. The numbered oblique cross-cuts are perpendicular to the arc and indicate the specific location of slices through proposed implant sites. *B,* Cross-sectional images corresponding to numbered slices on the axial image (*A*). Note how the buccal and lingual bone configuration and cortical thickness are demonstrated, as well as the location of the mental foramen in slice 32. (Courtesy of Dr. S. Brent Dove, University of Texas Dental School at San Antonio, Texas.)

ning tops were placed on the table, they would all be oriented with their north pole pointing upward. In our bodies this is not the case, for our spinning hydrogen nuclei are randomly oriented. This random orientation of spinning hydrogen nuclei is one of the essential elements in generating a magnetic resonance image. Two other essential elements are the placement of the patient's body (made mostly of hydrogen atoms) in an external magnetic field and the introduction of radiofrequency energy pulses.

The MR scanner is a cylindrical device into which the patient, lying on a specially designed table, is placed. The scanner surrounds the patient's body with powerful electromagnets. These electromagnets create an extremely strong external magnetic field that causes the randomly oriented spinning nuclei of hydrogen atoms in the patient's body to align, much like the spinning tops on a table. Just as the spinning tops on a table wobble as they fight the effects of gravity trying to knock them over, the spinning hydrogen nuclei wobble as they struggle against the external magnetic field to return to their randomly oriented state. The stronger the external magnetic field holding the hydrogen nuclei in alignment, the faster they wobble. Since the rate at which the hydrogen nuclei wobble is related to the strength of the external magnetic field surrounding the patient, this information can be used to tailor MR examinations to specific applications.

We now have a patient in the scanner and subjected to an external magnetic field of known strength, which results in a proportionate degree of alignment of the spinning hydrogen nuclei. This state of affairs is now intentionally disrupted when a radiofrequency energy pulse, timed to the same rate of wobble as the spinning hydrogen nuclei, knocks them out of alignment. Still in the scanner's magnetic field, the disrupted nuclei begin to realign within milliseconds. The realignment process emits distinctive radiofrequency signals, which are stored in a computer. Different tissues can be distinguished based on the rate at which their hydrogen nuclei realign and on the density or number of hydrogen atoms returning a signal. The computer transforms these data into an image based on the time it took the hydrogen nuclei to realign and on the number of hydrogen atoms sending a return signal.

Magnetic resonance imaging and computed tomography are often used as complementary studies. Magnetic resonance is superior for imaging soft tissues, because it takes advantage of the water content of tissues, and CT is best reserved for imaging bone. Although CT provides good quality images of soft tissue, the differentiation of one tissue from adjacent tissue(s) is much better with MR technology. Magnetic resonance imaging offers *enhanced soft tissue contrast* when compared with CT.

Another advantage of MR is known as *direct multiplanar imaging*. Using MRI technology, the plane through the region of the body to be examined is not limited by the position of the patient relative to the gantry, as in CT. The layer to be imaged by MR can be selected electronically, thus allowing direct imaging in the axial, sagittal, coronal, and oblique planes. Additionally, images of a preselected volume or area of tissue can be made directly.

Improved tissue contrast and multiplanar capabilities have made MR the imaging modality of choice for evaluating most head and neck soft tissue lesions, such as cysts and neoplasms, developmental anomalies, and inflammatory processes. Again, bony involvement is best assessed with CT.

Magnetic resonance imaging has proved to be superior for visualizing the

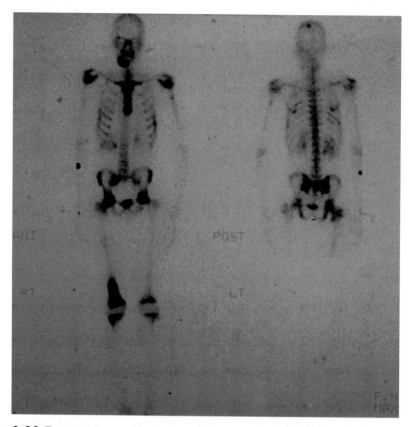

Figure 1-14. Bone scan image. The dark areas represent anatomical sites where the circulating radionuclide has been retained.

structures comprising the temporomandibular joints. Although CT gives excellent bone definition, it falls short in imaging internal joint anatomy, especially the articular disk. Computed tomography and MR images are presented in Chapter 8, along with other extraoral projections.

RADIONUCLIDE IMAGING

Thus far we have discussed x rays and radiofrequency emissions as the energy types that transfer patient data to the image receptor to create a picture. Radionuclide imaging uses still another form of energy, which is sometimes referred to as *internal source radiation*. Nuclear medicine techniques involve the intravenous injection of a radionuclide (radiopharmaceutical agent) into the bloodstream. Once the injected solution has become dispersed throughout the body, tissues exhibiting increased metabolic activity will retain more of the radionuclide than tissues functioning at a normal rate. This is because hyperactive tissues experience an increase in the amount of blood flowing through them, which in turn delivers more of the radiopharmaceutical agent to those tissues. After a period of time has elapsed (the half-life), specific to the radionuclide used, radiation is emitted from inside the patient, i.e., internal source radiation. The radionuclide is undergoing *radio-active decay.*

The image receptor is a specialized camera, called a *gamma camera,* that performs the function of a Geiger counter. The gamma camera detects the varying amounts of radiation being emitted from within the patient, and the computer translates the data into an image. Images resulting from a radionuclide scan are unique in appearance. Although many areas throughout the body will retain a quantity of the radiopharmaceutical agent and be imaged as a gray tone, the areas of hyperactivity will appear as dark or black. An intense, black image in the region of interest is often referred to as a "hot spot," and it represents increased circulation and increased radionuclide in the area (Fig. 1–14).

Radionuclide scans are often ordered to assess activity in bone, thyroid and salivary glands, liver, and brain. Increased activity in these tissues and organs can result from (1) primary or metastatic lesions of cancer; (2) infection such as osteomyelitis, tooth abscess, sinusitis; (3) inflammation accompanying arthritis, or salivary gland infection; or (4) any other situation resulting in increased circulation and/or metabolic activity.

Some of the more commonly used radionuclides are ^{99m}TcMDP (technetium medronate disodium), ^{99m}Tc polyphosphate, ^{99m}TcO$_4^-$ (pertechnetate), ^{67}Ga (gallium citrate), ^{125}I (iodine), and ^{18}F (fluorine). A dose of approximately 2.0 rad (20 milliGray, mGy) is administered during the average whole body bone scan.

REFERENCES

Brooks SL: Computed tomography. Dent Clin North Am 1993; 37(4):575–590.

Brooks SL, Miles DA: Advances in diagnostic imaging in dentistry. Dento Maxillofac Radiol 1993; 37(1):91–111.

Bushong SC: Special x-ray equipment and procedures. In Radiologic Science for Technologists: Physics, Biology, and Protection, 4th edition, p 308. St. Louis, CV Mosby, 1988.

Bushong SC: Digital x-ray imaging. In Radiologic Science for Technologists: Physics, Biology, and Protection, 4th edition, p 363. St. Louis, CV Mosby, 1988.

Bushong SC: Computed tomography. In Radiologic Science for Technologists: Physics, Biology, and Protection, 4th edition, p 385. St. Louis, CV Mosby, 1988.

Bushong SC: Physical principles of magnetic resonance imaging. In Radiologic Science for Technologists: Physics, Biology, and Protection, 4th edition, p 409. St. Louis, CV Mosby, 1988.

Bushong SC: Magnetic resonance equipment and images. In Radiologic Science for Technologists: Physics, Biology, and Protection, 4th edition, p 427. St. Louis, CV Mosby, 1988.

Cook LT, Giger ML, Wetzel LH, et al: Digitized film radiography. Invest Radiol 1989; 24:910–916.

Dagenais ME, Clark BG: Receiver operating characteristics of RadioVisioGraphy. Oral Surg Oral Med Oral Pathol 1995;79(2):238–245.

Dove SB: Digital imaging in dentistry. American Academy of Oral and Maxillofacial Radiology NEWSLETTER, Winter 1992; 19(1).

Dove SB, McDavid WD: A comparison of conventional intra-oral radiography and computer imaging techniques for the detection of proximal surface dental caries. Dento Maxillofac Radiol 1992; 21(3): 127–134.

Dove SB, McDavid WD: Digital panoramic and extraoral imaging. Dent Clin North Am 1993; 37(4):541–551.

Edwards MK: Magnetic resonance imaging of the head and neck. Dent Clin North Am 1993; 37(4):591–611.

Frederiksen NL: Specialized radiographic techniques. In Goaz PW, White SC: Oral Radiology: Principles and Interpretation, 3rd edition, p 266. St. Louis, CV Mosby, 1994.

Goaz PW, White SC: Extraoral radiographic examinations. In Oral Radiology: Principles and Interpretation, 3rd edition, p 227. St. Louis, CV Mosby, 1994.

Gratt BM: Panoramic radiography. In Goaz PW, White SC: Oral Radiology: Principles and Interpretation, 3rd edition, p 242. St. Louis, CV Mosby, 1994.

Grondahl HG, Grondahl K: Subtraction radiography for the diagnosis of periodontal bone lesions. Oral Surg Oral Med Oral Pathol 1983; 55:208–213.

Grondahl HG, Grondahl K, Webber RL: Influence of variation in projection geometry on the detectability of periodontal bone lesions. A comparison between subtraction radiography and conventional radiographic technique. J Clin Periodontol 1984; 11:411–420.

Horner K, Shearer AC, Walker A, et al: RadioVisioGraphy: An initial evaluation. Br Dent J 1990; 168:244–248.

Kassebaum DK, Nummikoski PV, Triplett RG, et al: Cross-sectional radiography for implant site assessment. Oral Surg Oral Med Oral Pathol 1990; 70(5):674–678.

Kundel HL, Revesz G: Lesion conspicuity, structured noise and film reader error. Am J Roentgenol 1976; 126:1233–1238.

McDavid WD, Dove SB, Welander U, et al: Direct digital extraoral radiography of the head and neck with a solid-state linear x-ray detector. Oral Surg Oral Med Oral Pathol 1992; 74:811–817.

McMillan JH, Huang HKB, Bramble JM, et al: Digital radiography. Invest Radiol 1989; 24:735–741.

Miles DA: Imaging using solid-state detectors. Dent Clin North Am 1993; 37(4):531–540.

Miles DA, Van Dis ML, Razmus TF: Plain film extraoral radiographic techniques. In Basic Principles of Oral and Maxillofacial Radiology, p 123. Philadelphia, WB Saunders, 1992.

Miles DA, Van Dis ML, Razmus TF: Advanced imaging modalities. In Basic Principles of Oral and Maxillofacial Radiology, p 185. Philadelphia, WB Saunders, 1992.

Mouyen R, Benz C, Sonnabend, et al: Presentation and physical evaluation of RadioVisioGraphy. Oral Surg Oral Med Oral Pathol 1989; 68:238–242.

Nelvig P, Wing K, Welander U: Sens-A-Ray: A new system for direct digital intraoral radiography. Oral Surg Oral Med Oral Pathol 1992; 74:818–823.

Ohki M, Okano T, Nakamura T: Factors determining the diagnostic accuracy of digitized conventional intraoral radiographs. Dento Maxillofac Radiol 1994; 23(2):77–82.

Razmus TF, Glass BJ, McDavid WD: Comparison of image layer location among panoramic machines of the same manufacturer. Oral Surg Oral Med Oral Pathol 1989;67:102–108.

Razzano MR, Bonner PJ: RadioVisioGraphy; Video imaging alters traditional approach to radiography. Compend Contin Educ Dent 1990; 11(6):398–400.

Reddy MS, Jeffcoat MK: Digital subtraction radiography. Dent Clin North Am 1993; 37(4):553–565.

Rethman M, Ruttiman V, O'Neal R, et al: Diagnosis of bone lesions by subtraction radiography. J Clin Periodontol 1985;56:324–329.

Revesz G, Kundel HL, Graber MA: The influence of structured noise on the detection of radiologic abnormalities. Invest Radiol 1974;9:479–486.

Schwarz MS, Rothman SLG, Chafetz N, et al: Computed tomography in dental implantation surgery. Dent Clin North Am 1989;33(4):555–597.

Tyndall DA, Kapa SF, Bagnell CP: Digital subtraction radiography for detecting cortical and cancellous bone changes in the periapical region. J Endodont 1990;16:173–178.

vander Stelt PF: Practical digital imaging: The future role of digital imaging in dentistry and in oral and maxillofacial radiology. American Academy of Oral and Maxillofacial Radiology NEWSLETTER, Winter 1994;21(1).

Zubery Y: Computerized image analysis in dentistry: Present status and future applications. Compend Contin Educ Dent 1993;8(11):964–973.

2

X RAYS—THEIR SOURCE AND BEHAVIOR

THOMAS F. RAZMUS

Electromagnetic Energies

Atomic Structure

The X-Ray Machine

The X-Ray Tube

X-Ray Production

X-Ray Interactions with Matter

Quality Assurance for Intraoral X-Ray Machines

Quality Assurance for Specialized X-Ray Machines

Chapter 2 discusses radiation physics as it applies to the nature, behavior, and generation of x rays, and how x rays interact with matter. The focus is on the production of x rays in a generic dental x-ray machine. The physical principles resulting in the production of x rays encompass atomic structure and interactions between subatomic particles. The force driving x-ray production is electricity. The controls on a dental x-ray machine control box can be used to vary the electrical energy supplied to the x-ray machine. The operator has the capability to "fine-tune" the energy of the x-ray beam, which in turn affects patient radiation dose and the characteristics of the resultant image. The interactions of x rays with matter are also subatomic in nature and analogous to the interactions that produce x rays, but with certain differences that will be discussed shortly. Matter is defined as anything that occupies space and has mass or weight.

When radiation energy passes through a biological entity, several things may happen to both the radiation and the biological material. *Excitation* of a biological atom or molecule is said to occur if the incident radiation causes an electron to be raised to a higher energy level without the loss of any electrons from the atom or molecule. If the incoming radiation has enough energy to eject an electron from the atom or molecule, resulting in a net positive charge on the atom or molecule, the radiation is called *ionizing radiation.* Ionizing radiation can be classed as *particulate* or *electromagnetic.* Particulate and electromagnetic radiations differ in the rate at which they transfer their energy to the medium through which they are passing. This is the concept of *linear energy transfer* (LET), which will be discussed in Chapter 4.

ELECTROMAGNETIC ENERGIES

Electromagnetic energy is composed of electric and magnetic fields. This group of energies consists of a *spectrum,* or range, of energy levels. These

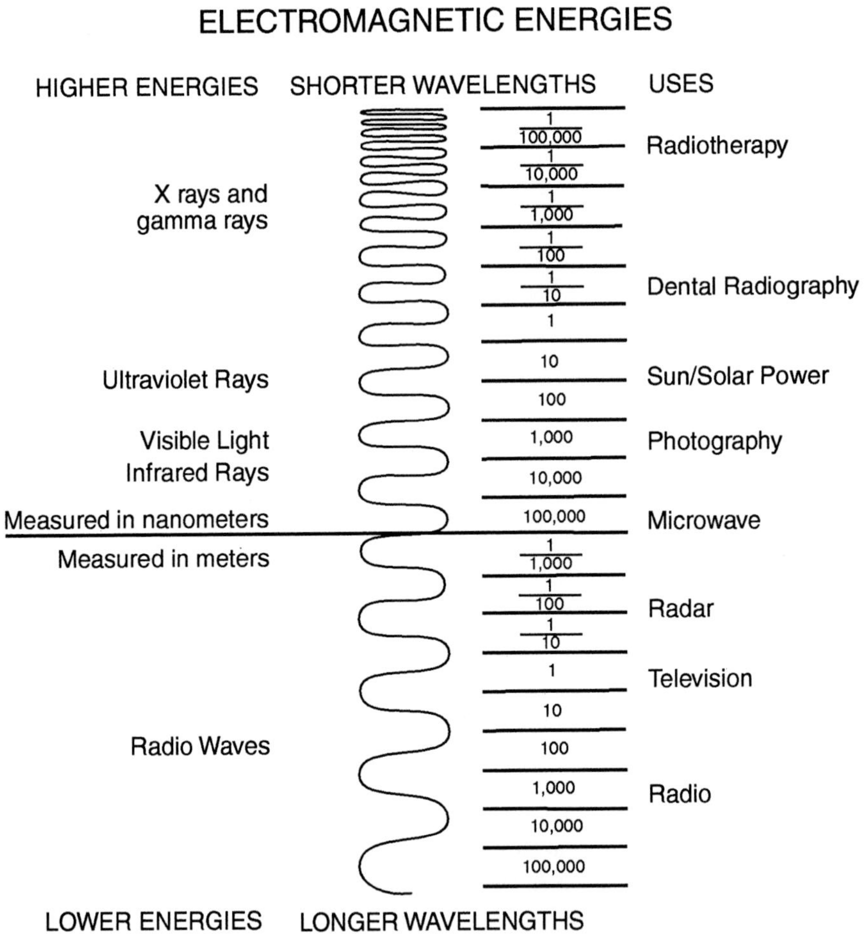

Figure 2-1. The spectrum, or range, of electromagnetic energies.

energies are propagated or transmitted through space (air) as *particles* and *waves*. Radiation physics terminology refers to this as the *particle concept* and *wave concept* of energy propagation. X rays are one type of electromagnetic energy (Fig. 2–1).

Energy propagated as a particle might be thought of as a discrete bundle of energy referred to as a *photon*. Calling to mind the space ship in a popular television series firing "photon torpedoes" at an alien spacecraft may help visualization of the photon concept of energy propagation. The photon carries the radiation energy in discrete, measurable units. The amount of energy carried by a photon depends upon the frequency and wavelength of the radiation and is referred to as *photon energy*. The particle or photon concept of x-ray propagation should not be confused with the classification of particulate ionizing radiations.

Ripples on a pond are a common wave form. Another common wave can be produced by tying a length of rope to a doorknob, taking hold of the free end, and "whipping" it. The harder you whip the free end, the more waves are produced between you and the doorknob. The more energy you put into the rope, the more waves result. The range of energy levels inherent in the electromagnetic spectrum, as well as within each energy type within the spectrum, is based on the concepts of *wavelength* and *frequency*.

Wavelength is the distance from the crest or trough of one wave to the crest or trough of the next wave. *Frequency* is the number of wavelengths traversing a given distance (Fig. 2–2). Energy characterized by long wavelengths will have fewer waves in a given distance compared with an energy form

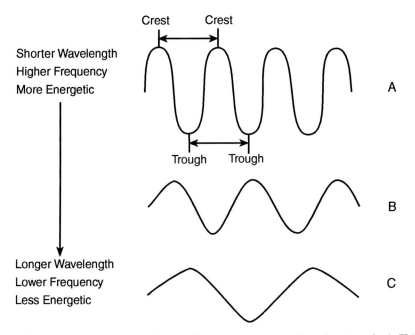

Figure 2–2. One wavelength is the distance from crest to crest, or trough to trough. *A,* This wave exhibits the highest frequency and shortest wavelength of the three waves illustrated, and it will possess the greatest energy. *B* and *C,* As the wavelength increases and the frequency decreases, energy will diminish.

having short wavelengths. The short wavelength energy will have a higher frequency than the long wavelength energy. Wavelength and frequency determine the *energy level* of the various types of electromagnetic energy. An x ray characterized by long wavelengths will have a lower frequency than a short wavelength x ray. The long wavelength, lower frequency x ray will be less energetic than the short wavelength, higher frequency x ray. The more energetic x ray is better able to penetrate the patient than the lower energy x ray. Each type of x ray will affect patient radiation dose and the radiographic image differently (Table 2–1).

Chapter 3 discusses how x-ray beam energy influences radiographic image contrast and density. Chapter 4 provides an explanation of how x-ray beam energy affects patient dose.

ATOMIC STRUCTURE

The simplest model of an atom portrays a small, dense, positively charged nucleus surrounded by negatively charged electrons orbiting in discrete energy levels designated as K, L, M, N, etc. (see Figs. 2–11, 2–12, 2–13). The number of electrons is equal to the number of positive charges on the nucleus. The positively charged nucleus exerts a pull, or *nuclear attraction,* on the negatively charged electrons. The strength of the nuclear attraction is greatest for electrons in the K-energy level since it is closest to the nucleus.

As electrons orbit the nucleus, their speed of travel tends to direct them in a straight line away from the nucleus (centrifugal force), but the nuclear attraction holds them in their orbit or energy level. The nuclear attraction is, therefore, referred to as the *electron-binding energy.* The electron-binding energy is *characteristic* for each energy level and for each chemical element.

Atoms are in a stable state by nature. Stability exists when each energy level is filled with its characteristic number of electrons. A vacancy in an energy level causes an unstable condition, necessitating a reaction to eliminate the vacancy. The vacancy is often eliminated by electrons from the next higher energy level falling into the space. Energy levels farther removed from the nucleus may also contribute an electron to fill a vacancy. The end result is a cascade of electrons toward the nucleus, resulting in energy levels closest to the nucleus being filled first. When an electron falls from one energy level to another, a characteristic amount of energy is given off. The amount of

Table 2–1. Characteristics of X-Ray Beam Energy Levels

Higher Energy	Lower Energy
Shorter wavelength	Longer wavelength
Higher frequency	Lower frequency
More penetrating	Less penetrating
Lower patient dose	Higher patient dose
Lower contrast image	Higher contrast image
Higher density image	Lower density image

energy is equal to the difference in electron-binding energies between the two levels involved and is *characteristic* for each chemical element. We will discuss this relative to the production of *characteristic radiation*. Characteristic radiation is generated in the x-ray tube during x-ray production and when x rays interact with matter.

Industry analyzes various materials with x rays possessing energy levels different from those used in dentistry and medicine. Medicine uses different energy levels of x rays depending upon whether the application is diagnostic or therapeutic. The energy exhibited by an x ray depends upon the chemical element from which the x ray was created and the energy expended to generate the x ray. Diagnostic images in dentistry and medicine result from the use of x rays within the *diagnostic energy range*. The chemical element used for dental diagnostic radiography is *tungsten*. Tungsten is used because its atomic number and subatomic structure are optimal for production of x rays in the diagnostic energy range. Tungsten has a high melting point, which allows it to withstand the extreme heat generated during x-ray production. The high ductility of tungsten allows it to be drawn into a fine wire, such as the cathode filament, without breaking. The machine components made of tungsten are located in the *x-ray tube*.

THE X-RAY MACHINE

The *x-ray machine* consists of the myriad of components from the electrical hookup or wall receptacle to the point where x rays exit the machine.

Structural Components

The *electrical cables* run inside the suspension arm and carry the power to generate x rays. The *suspension arm* allows for positioning the tubehead in proximity to the patient. The *yoke* is the U-shaped structure at the end of the suspension arm, which holds the tubehead. The *tubehead* is the heart of an intraoral x-ray machine; it is the structure that the operator handles when lining up the x-ray beam to make a radiograph. The tubehead contains the *x-ray tube* and two *transformers* surrounded by an *oil bath* (Fig. 2–3).

X-Ray Generating Components

The generation of x rays takes place in the x-ray tube and creates great amounts of heat. More than 99% of the energy expended to generate x rays is given off as heat, leaving less than 1% that is actually transformed into x-ray energy. The oil bath surrounding the x-ray tube dissipates this heat to the tubehead casing and into the operatory. Since anywhere from 70 thousand (70 kV) to 90 thousand (90 kV) volts of electricity are used to generate x rays, the oil bath also serves as an electrical insulator. Veteran operators will have experienced the cooling effect of the oil bath as the tubehead casing becomes warm after several radiographs are made in rapid succession.

X-ray machines cannot operate on standard voltages. A transformer is an

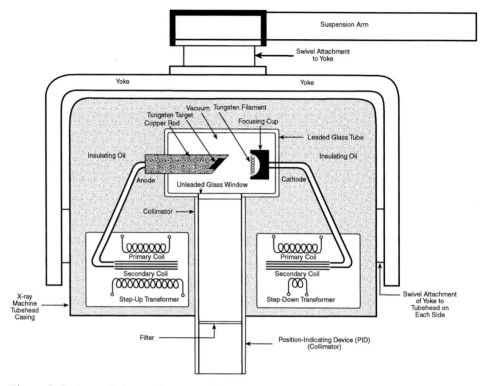

Figure 2–3. A generic intraoral x-ray machine tubehead and its major components. For orientation purposes, the reader should visit an operatory that houses an intraoral x-ray machine. This diagram is meant to illustrate a tubehead aimed at the floor and being viewed from the top of the machine tubehead casing. The reader is encouraged to refer to this diagram often while studying this and other chapters.

electrical device that changes the voltage of the incoming electric current. Inside the tubehead the two transformers "transform" the standard voltage as supplied by the electric company and deliver it to the x-ray tube. One of the two transformers is called a *step-up* transformer, and the other is a *step-down* transformer. The step-up transformer will increase the standard supplied voltage to 50 to 100 thousand volts (50 to 100 kV) in most intraoral machines. The step-up transformer creates the *high-voltage circuit* of the x-ray tube and is often referred to as the *tube current*. The standard voltage will be decreased to 8 to 12 volts by the step-down transformer, thus creating the *low-voltage circuit* of the x-ray tube. The *mA (milliampere) control* is used to manipulate the low-voltage circuit and the *kVp (kilovolt peak) control* is used to manipulate the high-voltage circuit.

Components That Control X-Ray Production and Affect the Resultant Image

The *control box* ideally should be situated behind a radiation-proof barrier, which is the location from which the operator will radiograph a patient (Fig. 2–4). A generic control box for an intraoral x-ray machine contains the

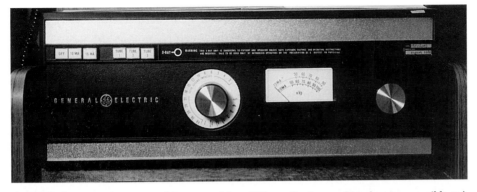

Figure 2–4. A typical x-ray machine control box. This particular machine has two possible mA settings in the upper left corner. The exposure timer is the round dial in the center. The kVp meter has two scales to match the kVp range to the mA selected. The dial on the right regulates an autotransformer to adjust the kVp setting.

exposure timer, exposure button, milliamperage (mA) control, and kilovolt peak (kVp) control (autotransformer). Some manufacturers do not provide the features to allow adjustment of the mA and/or kVp, and these controls will be absent from those machines.

The *exposure timer* is set by the operator to limit the length of time x rays will be generated when making a radiograph (Fig. 2–5). Since radiographic exposures require less than 1 second, timers are calibrated in fractions of a second. Calibrations may be in standard fractions of a second, decimal fractions of a second, or in impulses. All calibrations are based on the division of time into 60 increments.

> One hour = 60 minutes
> One minute = 60 seconds
> One second = 60 impulses

Figure 2–5. Enlargement of the exposure timer dial from Figure 2–4. Note that the most common timer settings used in intraoral radiography are represented in impulses and occupy most of the space on the dial. Most intraoral exposures are less than 1 second in duration—that is, less than 60 impulses.

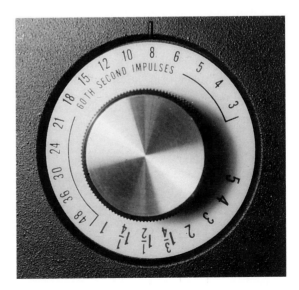

20 impulses = 20/60 second = 1/3 second = 0.33 second

The *exposure button* is called a "deadman" type of switch. The requirements for such a switch are that it trigger only one exposure each time it is pushed, and that it must be held down for the exposure to be completed. Most x-ray machines produce an audible beep or flashing light when the exposure is finished, signaling that the switch may be released.

The *mA control* determines the number of x rays generated during a given length of exposure time. Exposure time determines how long this number of x rays is allowed to leave the machine. Most intraoral x-ray machines that have an adjustable mA will offer the option of 10 mA or 15 mA.

Since exposure time and mA, each in its own way, affect the number of x rays exiting from the x-ray machine, they can be combined as a single factor called *milliamperage × seconds* (mAs). The main effect of exposure time(s), milliamperage (mA), or their combination as milliamperage × seconds (mAs) is on the *density* of the radiograph. *Density is defined as the overall darkness of the radiograph.* These exposure factors can be varied to maintain or change the density of a radiograph.

5 mA × 0.30 sec = 1.5 mAs

10 mA × 0.15 sec = 1.5 mAs

15 mA × 0.10 sec = 1.5 mAs

When a situation arises in which the original density of a radiograph must be maintained or changed, exposure time is the factor most easily adjusted. A common scenario is the need to increase or decrease exposure time to compensate for large or small patients, respectively, to maintain optimal radiographic density. Since exposure timers are calibrated in fractions of a second, it is possible to adjust density in small increments.

As mentioned earlier, the manufacturer may not provide a means by which to adjust the mA. If an mA control is available, the changes in density will be more profound than by using exposure time, because the mA can be changed only in increments of 5 mA—i.e., 5 mA, 10 mA, or 15 mA settings. If the unlikely situation arises in which adjusting the mA to maintain the original density of a radiograph is more appropriate, the operator should multiply the original exposure time by two or three for a decrease of every 5 mA, or divide the original exposure time by two or three for an increase of each 5 mA. Maintaining the original density of a radiograph while altering mA essentially requires one third to one half more or less exposure time for each decrease or increase of 5 mA, respectively. This procedure will maintain the original density of the radiograph, because the mAs, or total exposure, remains unchanged. Again, most manipulations of radiographic density will be managed by varying the exposure time alone.

ADDITIONAL EXAMPLES OF EXPOSURE TIME AND mAs MANIPULATIONS

1. To change an exposure time in seconds to an exposure time in impulses, **multiply** the number of seconds by 60, as shown:

Exposure time in seconds × 60 = exposure time in impulses

An example for timers calibrated in fractions of a second:

1/6 second = ? impulses
1/6 × 60 = 60/6 = 10 impulses

An example for timers calibrated in decimals of a second:

0.20 second = ? impulses
0.20 × 60 = 12 impulses

2. To change an exposure time in impulses to an exposure time in seconds, **divide** the number of impulses by 60, as shown:

Number of impulses / 60 = exposure time in seconds

An example for timers calibrated in fractions of a second:

12 impulses = ? seconds
12/60 = 1/5 second

An example for timers calibrated in decimals of a second:

6 impulses = ? seconds
6/60 = 1/10 = 0.10 second

3. To calculate milliampere-seconds (mAs), **multiply** the milliamperage (mA) setting by the exposure time (seconds), as shown:

mA × exposure time = mAs

For example,

10 mA and a 1/2-second exposure time
10 × 1/2 = 10/2 = 5 mAs

Or,

5 mA and a 2-second exposure time
5 × 2 = 10 mAs

4. To calculate the exposure time needed to arrive at a particular mAs, **divide** the mAs by the mA, as shown:

Exposure time = mAs / mA

For example,

10 mA and ? seconds = 20 mAs

20/10 = 2 seconds

Or,

5 mA and ? seconds = 10 mAs

10/5 = 2 seconds

5. To calculate the mA needed to arrive at a particular mAs, **divide** the mAs by the exposure time, as shown:

mA = mAs / exposure time

For example,

? mA and 2 seconds = 20 mAs

20/2 = 10 mA

Or,

? mA and 3 seconds = 30 mAs

30/3 = 10 mA

The Inverse Square Law and Radiographic Density

The number of x rays in the x-ray beam exiting the machine is referred to as the *quantity* of the beam. *Intensity* of an x-ray beam is determined by the number of x rays that actually interact with the patient and the film to create a radiographic image. Exposure time and mA (mAs) are used to alter beam quantity, which is directly related to beam intensity. Beam intensity has a direct effect on radiographic density; that is, the more x rays that hit the film, the greater the density of the resultant radiograph. In addition to the contributions of exposure time and mA to beam intensity and radiographic density, the *distance* from the x-ray source to the film also has a major influence. The *inverse square law* states that *beam intensity is inversely related to the square of the source-to-film distance (SFD)*. Changing the SFD alters the intensity of the beam or the number (quantity) of x rays that will pass through the patient and interact with the image receptor to create an image (Fig. 2–6). Changing the SFD will influence the density of the resultant radiograph. Following are two simple "**rules of thumb**" that can be applied

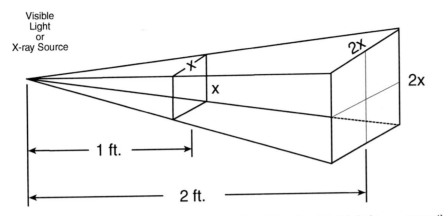

Figure 2–6. Diagram of the inverse square law. A given intensity of visible light or x rays will decrease to one fourth of its original quantity when the distance traversed is doubled.

to maintain the original radiographic density when a change of SFD is called for:

- **When the SFD is doubled, the original exposure time should be multiplied by four.**
- **When SFD is halved, the original exposure time should be divided by four, i.e., use one fourth the original exposure time.**

The following mathematical relationships may be used instead of the previously mentioned rules to calculate the new intensity or exposure time resulting from a change in the SFD.

Since the intensity of the x-ray beam is inversely proportional to the squares of the distances from the radiation source to the image receptor, the following formula can be used to calculate a new intensity at a new distance:

$$\frac{\textbf{Intensity}_1}{\textbf{Intensity}_2} = \frac{\textbf{(Distance}_2\textbf{)}^2}{\textbf{(Distance}_1\textbf{)}^2}$$

And,

Since beam intensity, radiographic density, and exposure time are directly related, the following formula can be used to calculate the new exposure time necessary to maintain the original density at a new distance. Exposure time is directly proportional to the squares of the distances from the radiation source to the image receptor, so:

$$\frac{\textbf{Exposure time}_1}{\textbf{Exposure time}_2} = \frac{\textbf{(Distance}_1\textbf{)}^2}{\textbf{(Distance}_2\textbf{)}^2}$$

For example:

If the exposure time at a source-to-film distance of 8 inches is 1.0 second, what will be the new exposure time needed to maintain the original radio-graphic density at 16 inches?

This problem may be solved by using the simple "rule of thumb" mentioned earlier, or by applying the formula relating exposure time to distance.

Applying the **rule of thumb** for maintaining density at a new SFD, simply **multiply the original exposure time by 4 when the SFD is doubled,** so: Exposure time at 16 inches will be 4.0 seconds.

Applying the **formula relating exposure time to distance:**

X = the new exposure time at 16 inches

So,

$$\frac{1 \text{ sec}}{X} = \frac{(8 \text{ in})^2}{(16 \text{ in})^2} = \frac{(1)^2}{(2)^2} = \frac{1}{4} = 4.0 \text{ sec}$$

Remember,

When changing (doubling) the source-to-receptor distance from 8 to 16 inches, **multiply** the exposure time by 4 to maintain the original radio-graphic density.

And,

When changing (reducing to one half) the source-to-receptor distance from 16 to 8 inches, **divide** the exposure time by 4 to maintain the original radio-graphic density.

X-Ray Beam Quality and Radiographic Contract

The *kVp control* is used to set the maximal energy of the x-ray beam. Some intraoral x-ray machines do not have an adjustable kVp. These are referred to as constant potential machines, and they operate at a constant 70 kVp. The kVp control on machines that allow adjustment is referred to as an *autotransformer*. The autotransformer functions as a rheostat and will deliver the voltage selected by the operator to the step-up transformer.

The energy of the x-ray beam affects its *penetrability,* also referred to as *quality*. The kVp setting is used to control the *contrast* in a radiographic image. *The contrast of a radiographic image can be defined as the number of shades of gray between the extremes of black and white.* A higher kVp beam (75 to 90 kVp) will produce an image with more shades of gray between black and white than a lower kVp beam (60 to 75 kVp). More shades of gray between black and white result in a gradual transition from the one extreme to the other, and this is referred to as *low contrast, or long-scale contrast.* When there are just a few shades of gray between black and white, this is known as *high contrast, or short-scale contrast.* A black and white checkered flag is an example of maximum high contrast or short-scale contrast.

Although kVp exerts its major influence on contrast, density is also affected.

A higher energy beam will penetrate the patient more completely and darken the image more than a lower energy beam. When it becomes necessary to alter contrast and maintain the original density of the image, exposure time must be adjusted to compensate for the change in penetrating ability of the beam at the new kVp setting. The following rules can be applied:

To increase contrast and maintain original density:
(1) Decrease the original kVp by 15 kVp
(2) Use 2 times the original exposure time.

To decrease contrast and maintain original density:
(1) Increase the original kVp by 15 kVp
(2) Use one half the original exposure time.

An additional factor that can alter the quality of an x-ray beam is *filtration.* Just before exiting from the tubehead, the x-ray beam must pass through a metal filter, usually made of aluminum. The purpose of this filter is to remove x rays of such low energy that they would not pass through the patient. These low-energy x rays would add needlessly to the radiation dose of the patient. This sort of filtration is installed by the manufacturer on all intraoral x-ray machines and is called *added filtration.*

At times there may be a need to increase the added filtration. Placing additional thicknesses of filter material over the manufacturer's filter will remove additional x rays from the lower energy range of the beam. The result is to raise the average (mean) energy of the beam, thus making it more penetrating. This procedure is sometimes followed to decrease patient dose while causing a minimal change in radiographic contrast or when changing imaging systems.

Another type of filtration present in all x-ray machines is *inherent filtration.* Inherent filtration results from the machine components through which the x rays must pass before exiting from the tubehead, excluding the manufacturer's added filtration. These components are the unleaded glass window of the x-ray tube and the oil bath surrounding the tube. The combination of added and inherent filtration results in *total filtration.* The specific thickness of total filtration required depends upon the maximal operating kVp of the particular machine.

1.5 mm filtration for less than 70 kVp
2.5 mm filtration for 70 kVp or more

The x-ray machine *collimator,* or *position-indicating device (PID),* is the round or rectangular device attached to the tubehead (see Figs. 2–3, 2–7; also see Figs. 4–8, 4–9). After x rays leave the x-ray tube where they are generated, they pass through the filters just discussed and exit from the tubehead to pass through the collimator, or PID. The collimator, or PID, serves to shape the x-ray beam that will expose the patient and to help the operator aim the beam at the structures of interest.

Collimators, or position-indicating devices can be made of plastic, lead-lined plastic, or aluminum, and they are available in different standard

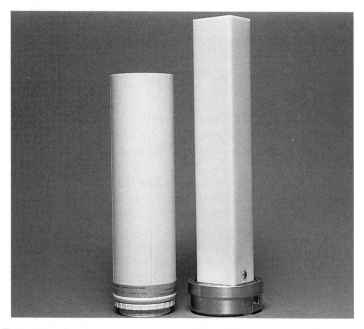

Figure 2–7. Round and rectangular collimators. These devices screw onto the machine housing. They shape the diverging x-ray beam after it exits the tubehead and provide a means for aiming the primary beam.

lengths. In the interest of keeping the radiation dose to the patient as low as possible, long, rectangular collimation is recommended.

THE X-RAY TUBE

Discussion of the components and concepts in previous sections was essential to developing an understanding of x-ray tube function and design. This section discusses how these components interface with the x-ray tube and result in x-ray production.

The average *x-ray tube* (see Fig. 2–3) in an intraoral machine is a cylindrical device approximately 3.0 inches (7.5 cm) in length, with a diameter of approximately 0.5 inch (1.25 cm). The tube is oriented perpendicular to the collimator and usually is located in the back half of the tubehead. The tube is made of *leaded glass,* except for a small area facing the collimator. This area of the tube, which is not leaded, is referred to as the *window* and is the only place generated x rays can exit from the tube. The window is oriented so that the x rays will exit from the tubehead through the filters (added filtration) and then be shaped by the collimator prior to exposing the patient. The atmosphere inside the tube is a *vacuum.* The process of x-ray production requires the movement and interaction of free tungsten electrons within the tube; any gas molecules present would interfere with the process.

Each end of the tube is an electrical terminal: one end is positive, called the *anode*; the other is negative, called the *cathode.* Be careful not to confuse similar terms used in chemistry, in which a cation is positive and an anion is negative. The anode and the cathode contain the tungsten components that will be active in x-ray production. The low-voltage circuit and mA control are associated with the cathode. The kVp control and the high-voltage circuit (tube current) affect the energy of the x rays produced at the anode.

The cathode will be discussed before the anode because the cathode is responsible for the number of free tungsten electrons available to generate x rays at the anode. The two major components of the cathode are the *filament* and the *focusing cup*. The filament is a tiny coil of tungsten less than 1 millimeter in diameter and not much more than one quarter of an inch in length. The focusing cup is made of molybdenum, and the filament spans the open end of the cup. The open end of the focusing cup faces the anode. The filament supplies the tungsten electrons for x-ray production, and the focusing cup "aims" the tungsten electron "stream" at the target on the anode.

When the exposure button is held down, the tungsten filament of the cathode is heated to glow "red-hot." Recall that the electrical current flowing through the cathode filament is the low-voltage circuit supplied by the step-down transformer and the mA control. The electrons near the surface of the filament are actually boiling from its surface when it has reached operating temperature, thus producing an *electron cloud* around the filament. The higher the mA, the higher the temperature of the filament and the more electrons will boil from the filament. The tungsten electrons in this cloud are temporarily free from the filament and therefore available for x-ray production. This process is referred to as *thermionic emission* (Fig. 2–8).

Therm: heating
-ionic: electrons
emission: "freed" from the filament

As the cathode filament is heating, the kVp control setting determines the strength of an electrostatic attraction from the cathode to the anode. The

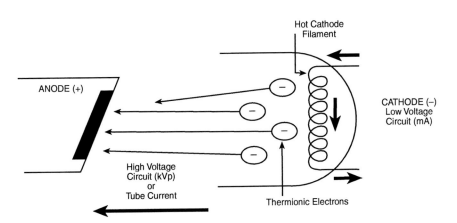

Figure 2–8. The low-voltage circuit directs current through the cathode filament. The filament becomes red-hot and releases electrons from its surface by thermionic emission. The mA control regulates the strength of the current flowing through the filament, the temperature of the filament, and the number of electrons released. The strength of the current through the high-voltage circuit or tube current is regulated by the kVp control. Tube current is flowing when thermionic electrons are moving across the tube vacuum from the cathode to the anode. The maximum speed of electrons across the vacuum is determined by the kVp setting.

purpose of this attractive force is to pull "free" electrons from the cloud around the filament and across the vacuum to the anode. An electrical cable connection to the end of the copper rod completes the route for the high-voltage circuit, or *tube current*. When electrons are moving across the vacuum from the cathode to the anode, the high-voltage circuit is operating and tube current is flowing (see Fig. 2–8). Tube current can "flow" only from the cathode to the anode for the x-ray tube to function. For this to occur, the x-ray tube must convert the alternating current (AC) supplied to it by the step-up transformer into a form of direct current (DC).

The standard electricity supplied to an x-ray machine is AC. Basically, alternating current flows in opposite directions 120 times per second. Direct current, on the other hand, does not change its direction. Voltage supplied as AC will cycle through a positive phase, to zero, and then through a negative phase and back to zero 60 times per second (60 cycles per second). The current in the positive phase flows in one direction, and the current in the negative phase flows in the opposite direction. *Rectification* is the process of converting AC to DC. The x-ray tube functions as a *rectifier* by using only the positive phase of the alternating current cycle. The positive phase of the alternating current functions as the tube current. This results in electrons flowing only from the cathode to the anode in impulses that occur 60 times per second. These x-ray machines are referred to as *self-rectified*. This phenomenon accounts for exposure timers being calibrated as they are, i.e., in fractions of a second (Fig. 2–9).

Variations in tube design have resulted in the production of *constant potential* and *full-wave rectified* x-ray machines. Constant potential machines incorporate a step-up transformer capable of amplifying standard AC of 60 cycles per second to 800 or more cycles per second. The extremely high frequency allows the amplified AC to act like a direct current. Full-wave rectification allows both the positive and negative phases of the alternating current to generate x rays. Intraoral x-ray machines are either self-rectified or constant potential units.

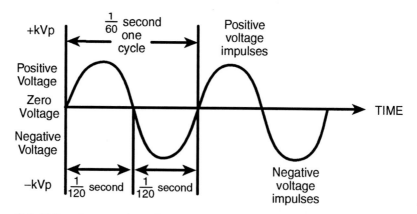

Figure 2–9. Voltage between the cathode and anode. Only the positive voltage impulses of each AC cycle are used in self-rectified x-ray machines. Note that the tube current voltage cycles from zero to the maximum (+ kVp) and then back to zero. This voltage fluctuation results in thermionic electrons being accelerated at different rates across the vacuum from the cathode to the anode, colliding with the anode target with varying intensity, and generating x rays of different energy levels.

The anode *target* is composed of a wafer of tungsten embedded in the end of the copper rod (see Fig. 2–3). The copper rod is no larger in diameter than a typical pencil, and it is 1.0 to 1.5 inches in length. The *tungsten target* wafer may be a square or rectangle of 2.0 to 3.0 mm on a side and 1.0 to 1.5 mm thick. As mentioned earlier, the generation of x rays creates a large amount of heat that is dissipated to the room atmosphere by the oil bath and tube housing. The source of the heat is within the tungsten target wafer. The purpose of the copper rod is to transfer the heat from the tungsten wafer to the oil bath.

The entire surface of the tungsten wafer is not involved in x-ray production. A small area near the center of the wafer, called the *focal spot,* is where x rays are produced, while the rest of the wafer aids in transferring heat to the copper rod. In addition to being the source of x rays, the focal spot has a major effect on image sharpness. The smaller the focal spot, within practical limits, the sharper the image. The size of the focal spot is determined by the manufacturer. Recall that the purpose of the molybdenum focusing cup is to direct the cathode electron stream at the focal spot.

The end of the copper rod positions the target wafer at an angle of 20° to the cathode filament (Fig. 2–10). This angulation causes the cathode electron stream to interact with a larger surface area of the target, as well as to direct most of the generated x rays toward the window of the x-ray tube. The angle results in variations of the shape and size of the focal spot, depending on whether it is viewed from the cathode or through the collimator. The focal spot seen from the cathode covers a larger area and is called the *actual focal spot.* This is the area upon which the stream of cathode electrons will make an impact. The larger surface area provides for greater x-ray production and heat dissipation. Looking through the collimator and window of the x-ray

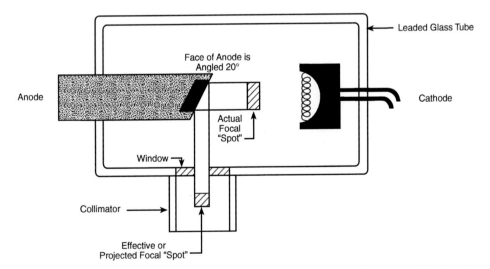

Figure 2-10. Application of the Benson line-focus principle results in placement of the face of the anode at an angle of 20° to the cathode, producing an effective or projected focal spot that will be smaller than the actual focal spot. The larger actual focal spot allows a greater area of the target to be exposed to the stream of thermionic electrons from the cathode, which enhances x-ray production and facilitates heat dissipation. The smaller projected focal spot maximizes image sharpness.

tube reveals a smaller focal spot known as the *effective* or *projected focal spot,* which is responsible for image production. Recall that a smaller focal spot will create a sharper image. The Benson line-focus principle prescribes placement of the face of the anode at an angle of 20°, which results in (1) a larger actual focal spot for more efficient x-ray generation and heat dissipation, and (2) a smaller effective or projected focal spot for maximal image sharpness.

X-RAY PRODUCTION

An x-ray beam contains many different levels of energy and thus is referred to as a *heterogeneous* beam. The beam emerging from the collimator is called the *primary,* or *useful,* beam. The center of the primary or useful beam is called the *central ray,* and it is designated to indicate the intended direction of the beam.

The positive voltage phase of the alternating current cycles from zero to a maximum voltage as set by the kVp control. The "p" in kVp refers to "peak" or maximal voltage. Peak kilovoltage exerts the maximal attractive force on the cathode tungsten electrons freed by thermionic emission. The strength of this electrical attraction varies from zero to a maximum and is directly related to the cycling AC voltage. The greater the maximal electrical attraction, the faster cathode electrons travel and the harder they "crash" into the tungsten target. Kilovolt peak determines the maximal speed of electrons traversing the vacuum, the maximal force of impact with the target, and maximal energy in the resultant x-ray beam.

The heterogeneous nature of the x-ray beam is composed of two specific types of x-ray radiation: *Bremsstrahlung radiation* (general or braking radiation) and *characteristic radiation.* Impacting cathode electrons will interact in several different ways with the electrons and nuclei of tungsten atoms in the target to produce these two fundamental types of x radiation.

Bremsstrahlung radiation results from interactions between incident cathode electrons and nuclei of tungsten atoms in the target. These interactions occur through the following mechanisms: (1) a direct hit on a tungsten nucleus in the target by an incident cathode electron, and (2) an incident cathode electron passing very near the nucleus of a tungsten atom in the target (Fig. 2–11).

A direct hit on a nucleus results in the fast-moving cathode electron giving up all its energy of motion (kinetic energy) in the collision. The electron's motion-energy is transformed into an x-ray photon with energy nearly equal to the kinetic energy possessed by the cathode electron at the time of impact. The mechanism of direct hits contributes a range of x-ray energies to the resultant beam, because each incident cathode electron has an impact with a force dependent on its speed at impact. The speed at impact depends upon where the electron was subjected to the attractive force from cathode to anode along the voltage continuum from zero to the kVp setting.

The majority of incident cathode electrons generate x rays by the second mechanism, which is much more complex than the first. The mechanism of "near hits" contributes spectral characteristics to the beam, depending upon (1) the speed of the cathode electron at impact, and (2) the proximity at which the incident electron passes the nucleus of a tungsten atom in the target. The

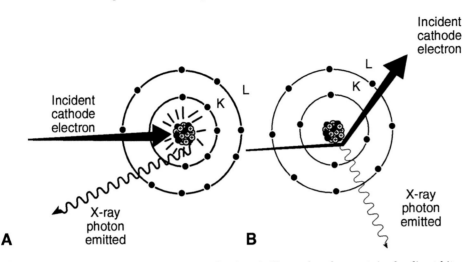

Figure 2–11. Bremsstrahlung radiation production. *A,* The nucleus has sustained a direct hit by a thermionic electron from the cathode. The incident electron has given all its energy to the reaction and ceases to exist. An x-ray photon has been emitted that has energy nearly equal to the kinetic energy of the cathode electron at impact. *B,* A thermionic electron has passed very near the nucleus. The electron's speed has been slowed and its direction changed by the electrostatic nuclear attraction. A photon of radiation was emitted. The incident electron will continue in a different direction at a speed proportional to its remaining kinetic energy.

positively charged nucleus attracts the passing, negatively charged electron, whereas the kinetic energy of the fast-moving electron tends to carry it past the nucleus. The combination of these two forces results in the incident electron being slowed and its direction being changed. The slowing of the electron constitutes a *braking effect.* An x-ray photon equal in energy to the lost kinetic energy is generated. An infinite variety of interactions is possible. Bremsstrahlung radiation not only accounts for the spectral characteristics of the beam but also contributes the major percentage of x-ray photons to the beam.

Characteristic radiation contributes a very small percentage of the energy to the x-ray beam (Fig. 2–12). The energy of the characteristic radiation will be equivalent to the difference in electron-binding energy between the two energy levels involved, as discussed earlier. This type of radiation occurs in small amounts because it requires incident cathode electrons to interact only with K- and L-shell electrons in tungsten target atoms to create useful x rays in the diagnostic energy range.

A vacancy results when an incident cathode electron knocks an orbiting K- or L-shell electron from its shell. An electron from a higher energy level, usually the next higher level, will move closer to the nucleus and fill the vacancy. The difference in electron-binding energy between the two energy levels is the energy of the resultant x-ray photon. This type of radiation is called characteristic because the photon energy (the difference between binding energies) will be characteristic of the chemical element involved.

X-RAY INTERACTIONS WITH MATTER

X-ray photons will interact with nuclei and orbiting electrons of atoms of matter in much the same way as cathode electrons interact with tungsten

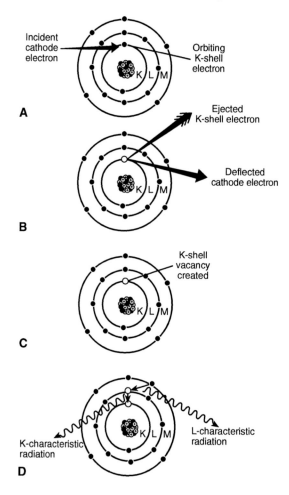

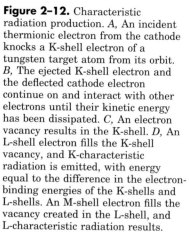

Figure 2-12. Characteristic radiation production. *A,* An incident thermionic electron from the cathode knocks a K-shell electron of a tungsten target atom from its orbit. *B,* The ejected K-shell electron and the deflected cathode electron continue on and interact with other electrons until their kinetic energy has been dissipated. *C,* An electron vacancy results in the K-shell. *D,* An L-shell electron fills the K-shell vacancy, and K-characteristic radiation is emitted, with energy equal to the difference in the electron-binding energies of the K-shells and L-shells. An M-shell electron fills the vacancy created in the L-shell, and L-characteristic radiation results.

nuclei and electrons in the target of the x-ray tube. When x radiation interacts with matter, some or all of its energy is lost, and a less energetic level of radiation emerges from the matter. The absorption of some or all of the energy of an x-ray beam as it passes through an object is called *attenuation,* and it is affected by the atomic number or density of the object, the thickness of the object, and the energy of the x-ray beam. Denser or higher atomic number structures within a patient, such as teeth and bone, will absorb or attenuate more of the energy from the beam than less dense or lower atomic number components, such as muscle and skin.

The x-ray beam that emerges from the patient will consist of a pattern of varying energy intensities, as a result of variable attenuation by patient structures. The emerging beam is composed of what remains of the original incident beam after having been attenuated by the patient's anatomical structures. This remaining beam is called the *remnant beam* or *remnant radiation.* The varying energy intensities in the remnant beam will interact with the image receptor to create an image. The image will be composed of darker areas, referred to as *radiolucent,* and lighter areas, designated as *radiopaque.* Patient structures that have attenuated more of the incident beam will generate the lighter or radiopaque objects in the image, because fewer x rays remained to interact with the image receptor. The radiolucent or darker areas of the image resulted from less attenuation of the beam by the less dense structures in the patient, thus allowing more x rays to interact with the image receptor.

An incident x-ray beam with higher energy or higher kVp will tend to pass more uniformly through any given patient, resulting in less variation in attenuation by the patient's anatomical structures. A higher energy beam will be less affected by the density or thickness of the structures through which it passes and will produce an image with many shades of gray between the extremes of black and white. Such an image is said to exhibit low contrast or long scale contrast. This type of image contrast is useful for detecting subtle changes in alveolar bone and may demonstrate other structures such as calculus, salivary stones, and even soft tissue outlines.

A lower energy or lower kVp beam will be more affected by object density (atomic number) and thickness. A lower kVp beam will produce an image with few shades of gray between the extremes of black and white and can be described as having high contrast or short scale contrast. High contrast images are useful for detecting early changes in high atomic number structures such as enamel, i.e., detecting early interproximal caries and following caries progression.

An x-ray photon can interact with matter in five basic ways:

1. Coherent or unmodified scattering
2. Photoelectric reaction or effect
3. Compton scattering
4. Pair production
5. Photodisintegration

The last two interactions do not occur in the diagnostic energy range and have no importance in diagnostic radiology.

Coherent or *unmodified scattering* occurs when a low energy x-ray photon passes close by an atom of matter and causes the atom to vibrate. No x-ray energy is transferred to the atom and no damage is done. The only effect is a change in direction of the x ray, thus the alternate name unmodified scattering.

The *photoelectric effect* is a relatively complex interaction resulting in the production of characteristic radiation, a negative ion (photoelectron) and a positive ion (Fig. 2–13). Recall that stable atoms are electrically balanced. A negative ion has an excess negative charge of one or more extra electrons; a positive ion has a deficiency of one or more electrons and a relative positive charge. Both these ions are unstable and can react with other ions, atoms, or molecules. The formation of unstable, reactive compounds called *free radicals* is the basis of radiation damage to living organisms.

Our earlier discussion of K- and L- characteristic radiation production in the x-ray tube is applicable here. The photoelectric effect occurs when an incident x-ray photon having a little more energy than a K-shell electron knocks one of these electrons from its energy level. Keep in mind that these are now K-shell electrons of some living tissue (matter) and not tungsten target atoms, as discussed earlier. Ejection of the K-shell electron by the x-ray photon requires the use of most of its energy to overcome the binding

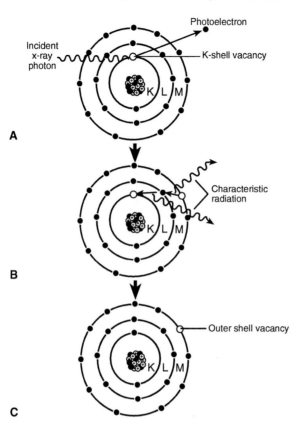

Figure 2–13. The photoelectric effect or interaction. *A,* An incident x-ray photon interacts with an atom of matter, and a K-shell electron is knocked from its orbit. This ejected electron is now called a photoelectron. *B,* Characteristic radiation is generated. *C,* The atom of matter has a deficiency of one electron and a net positive charge.

energy of the electron. Any remaining photon energy is transformed into kinetic energy to propel the K-shell electron away from its atom. The incident photon no longer exists. Thus far the reaction has produced (1) a negative ion, i.e., the ejected K-shell electron now called a *photoelectron,* and (2) a positive ion, the original atom deficient of one electron.

The third product of the photoelectric reaction, characteristic radiation, occurs by the same mechanism as discussed for radiation production in the x-ray tube. Radiation having energy characteristic of the element being irradiated will be emitted when electrons from a higher energy level move to fill the vacancy in the K-shell. These electrons usually come from the adjacent L-shell, occasionally the M-shell, and rarely from shells at a greater distance from the nucleus. *Characteristic radiation results from the movement of electrons within an atom. The x-ray energy emitted is characteristic of the element irradiated, i.e., calcium in bone, enamel, dentin, and so on.*

Scatter in diagnostic radiology results when the primary x-ray beam is deflected along its path to the image receptor (film, CCD, and so on) but ultimately reaches the receptor. A scattered photon gathers erroneous information and imparts energy to the patient along its path to the receptor. Scatter results in a higher dose to the patient and in loss of information from the image. *Compton scattering* accounts for most of the scatter in diagnostic radiology (Fig. 2–14).

Recall that characteristic radiation involves inner shell electrons that are

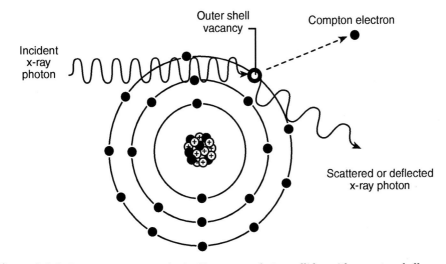

Figure 2–14. Compton scattering. An incident x-ray photon collides with an outer shell electron of an atom of matter. The electron is knocked from the atom and is designated as a "Compton" electron. The x-ray photon continues in a different direction with its remaining energy.

tightly bound in their orbit by a strong nuclear attraction and high electron-binding energy. Compton scattering, on the other hand, occurs when an x-ray photon collides with a loosely bound outer shell electron and knocks it out of its orbit. The colliding photon gives up part of its kinetic energy to dislodge the orbiting electron and then continues on in a different direction with slightly less energy. The photon will interact with other atoms until its energy is depleted or it reaches the image receptor. The "freed" electron is called a "Compton electron."

QUALITY ASSURANCE FOR INTRAORAL X-RAY MACHINES

A quality assurance (QA) program consists of specific tests, documentation of the results, and correction of problems or potential problems demonstrated by the test results to assure that a facility is producing high-quality radiographs in a consistent manner, at minimal cost to the patient and the facility, while exposing the patient and the employees to a minimal dose of radiation. The following discussion will address QA tests for intraoral x-ray machines. Quality assurance tests for the darkroom and film processing will be covered in a later chapter. A Quality Assurance Log Book should be kept for all tests performed and data collected.

X-Ray Machine Output Test

The *output* of an x-ray machine is the amount of radiation exposure it produces in air at a specific distance from the radiation source to the measuring instrument. This distance might be measured from the x-ray source to the skin surface if a patient were involved. The *x-ray machine output test* is used to monitor the reproducibility of radiation output by an x-ray machine. A *dosimeter* is the instrument used to measure the radiation coming from the machine. Several exposure readings are made while the exposure factors (mA, kVp, exposure time) and the source to instrument distance are held constant. The difference between the smallest and largest output readings should not exceed 10%. A difference greater than 10% indicates that the unit should be inspected by a service technician.

Kilovoltage Peak (kVp) Test

Kilovoltage (kV) is the tube current or flow of electrons across the vacuum in the x-ray tube. The kV selected on the control box and the tube current should always be the same. Inconsistency between the kVp setting and the actual tube current will affect contrast and, to a lesser extent, the density of the resultant radiograph. *Kilovoltage peak (kVp)* can be evaluated using instrumentation or a modified film cassette, commercially available as the Wisconsin kVp Test Cassette (Radiation Measurements, Inc., Middleton, Wisconsin).

Readings from the kilovoltage peak test instrument should be within the specifications provided by the manufacturer. The Wisconsin kVp Test Cassette produces a series of circular images on a piece of film, the densities of which are transferred to a calibration curve. The resulting plot is compared with a standardized plot provided by the manufacturer of the cassette. Results from either test method that fall outside the tolerance limits set by the test device manufacturer should prompt the operator to have the x-ray machine evaluated by trained service personnel.

Half-Value Layer Test

The HVL test is a modification of the x-ray machine output test. Rather than simply measuring the output of the machine, the HVL test uses the dosimeter readings to assess the penetrability of the beam. The HVL test determines the thickness of added aluminum filtration necessary to reduce the output of the machine by half. This is accomplished by placing aluminum filters in front of the beam until a thickness is reached that cuts the beam's intensity by half. These tests are run at 90 kVp, and the output is measured using a dosimeter. When an x-ray machine is assembled, it is the manufacturer's responsibility to ensure that the machine will meet the requirement of having a half-value layer equivalent to 2.5 mm of aluminum.

Exposure Timer Test

The exposure timer limits the time span over which x rays will be generated, thereby affecting density of the resultant radiograph. The exposure time set for the x-ray machine should agree with what is measured by a test device. The test device may be an electronic meter that gives the length of the exposure as a digital readout, or it may be a device called a *spinning top.* Electronic evaluation is accomplished by using exposure factors recommended by the manufacturer of the test instrument and making sure that test results fall within the tolerance limits provided by the manufacturer of the test meter.

The spinning top is a simple but effective tool for demonstrating the number of impulses that an x-ray machine is generating. Testing with the spinning top should be performed at a timer setting commonly used in the office. An occlusal film, with its solid white or film side facing up, is placed on a flat surface, and the top is spun on the surface of the film packet. The top should be spinning fast enough to remain vertical for several seconds. While the top is spinning, the collimator is brought directly above it and aligned perpendicular to the film and the exposure is made. A circular array of dots is imaged. The number of dots should correspond to the number of impulses set on the exposure timer. Timers calibrated in decimals or fractions of a second will need their values converted to impulses.

Milliamperage Test

Milliamperage, along with exposure time, is responsible for the quantity and intensity of the x-ray beam and for the density of the resultant radiograph. Recall that exposure time and mA work together as the combined factor of mAs to produce radiographic density. Milliamperage is tested by using a predetermined kVp, such as 80, and a constant mAs incorporating different combinations of mA and exposure time.

Using 80 kVp
15 mA and 24 impulses = 360 mAs
10 mA and 36 impulses = 360 mAs
5 mA and 72 impulses = 360 mAs

Since all the foregoing combinations result in the same mAs, the resultant test radiographs should have the same density. The test is performed by placing a piece of intraoral film on a flat surface with its white or radiation-sensitive side facing upward. An aluminum step wedge is positioned on top of the film, the end of the collimator is brought approximately an inch from the top of the step wedge and perpendicular to the film, and the exposure is made using one of the preceding factor combinations at 80 kVp. This is repeated for each factor combination. The three resulting films should appear identical, because the same mAs and kVp were used to create the images. The films should be compared side-by-side, and if the density of the step images vary by more than two steps, the machine should be inspected by a service representative.

Focal Spot Size Test

The focal spot is the small area of the tungsten target where x rays are generated. As an x-ray tube is used, the extreme temperatures can cause the surface of the target to deteriorate as a result of pitting. This results in an increase in the size of the actual focal spot. The size of the focal spot has a major effect on image sharpness. If the actual focal spot increases in size, the projected focal spot will do likewise, and its ability to define small structures will be decreased.

Within the limits set by the manufacturer, focal spot size varies along with changes of mA and kVp settings. Consequently, periodic determinations of the focal spot size should be made at the same mA and kVp. Machines that have been in service for less than 6 years should have their focal spot size monitored yearly. Older units require inspection at 6-month intervals. These tests are best performed by trained personnel.

Beam Alignment and Collimation Test

Consistent exposure of a precise area of the patient and image receptor is possible only if the central ray of the x-ray beam travels in the center of the collimator. Achievement of this situation requires that the x-ray tube within the machine housing be aligned with the aperture of the lead diaphragm where the x rays exit from the tubehead. Misalignment will result in the central ray traveling a diagonal path through the collimator. Unproductive irradiation of the patient will occur if the beam, the collimator, or both are not aligned. Collimation refers to the final shaping of the beam before it leaves the confines of the collimator, after which it will diverge according to the inverse square law. The diameter of the beam at the end of a round collimator should not exceed 7.0 cm (2.75 in). A rectangular collimator limits the size of the beam to just slightly greater than a number 2 intraoral film packet. These tests are best performed by a service technician.

Suspension Arm Stability Testing

Motion unsharpness can degrade the radiographic image if an unstable suspension arm allows movement of the tubehead to occur. Most suspension arms are stabilized by adjustable hydraulic and coil spring dampeners. These adjustments are usually included in the "trouble-shooting" section of the equipment owner's manual.

QUALITY ASSURANCE FOR SPECIALIZED X-RAY MACHINES

Panoramic and tomographic machines both require the synchronization and alignment of a complex mechanical system. Failure to achieve these requirements may result in an improperly located and/or shaped panoramic image layer, or a tomographic slice that is erroneously located or not of the expected thickness. Both scenarios will result in nondiagnostic information and unproductive irradiation of the patient.

The QA requirements for these types of machines are also unique. Radiation output can be measured by affixing a dosimeter to the end of the collimator. Total output is determined for the duration of the machine excursion. Exposure time is related to excursion time as well.

Image distortions may occur if the machine components responsible for image layer placement and thickness are not synchronized. Wear and tear of moving parts may be at fault: gears and pulleys may be worn; cables may be loose. If consistent anatomical image distortions have been observed in several consecutive radiographs, calculations of the depth and thickness of tomographic layers have been confirmed to be accurate, and the patients have been properly positioned, a malfunction or misalignment of the machine components should be suspected. Consistent anatomical image distortions not related to technique-specific errors or artifacts suggest that the machine may need to be calibrated, and a qualified service technician should be consulted.

REFERENCES

Bushong SC: Concepts of radiation. In Radiologic Science for Technologists: Physics, Biology, and Protection, 4th edition, p 1. St. Louis, CV Mosby, 1988.

Bushong SC: The atom. In Radiologic Science for Technologists: Physics, Biology, and Protection, 4th edition, p 30. St. Louis, CV Mosby, 1988.

Bushong SC: Electromagnetic radiation. In Radiologic Science for Technologists: Physics, Biology, and Protection, 4th edition, p 52. St. Louis, CV Mosby, 1988.

Bushong SC: Electromagnetism. In Radiologic Science for Technologists: Physics, Biology, and Protection, 4th edition, p 88. St. Louis, CV Mosby, 1988.

Bushong SC: The x-ray machine. In Radiologic Science for Technologists: Physics, Biology, and Protection, 4th edition, p 106. St. Louis, CV Mosby, 1988.

Bushong SC: X-ray production. In Radiologic Science for Technologists: Physics, Biology, and Protection, 4th edition, p 138. St. Louis, CV Mosby, 1988.

Bushong SC: X-ray interaction with matter. In Radiologic Science for Technologists: Physics, Biology, and Protection, 4th edition, p 156. St. Louis, CV Mosby, 1988.

Bushong SC: X-ray emission. In Radiologic Science for Technologists: Physics, Biology, and Protection, 4th edition, p 173. St. Louis, CV Mosby, 1988.

Bushong SC: Beam-restricting devices. In Radiologic Science for Technologists: Physics, Biology, and Protection, 4th edition, p 182. St. Louis, CV Mosby, 1988.

Hall EJ: The physics and chemistry of radiation absorption. In Radiobiology for the Radiologist, 3rd edition, p 1. Philadelphia, JB Lippincott, 1988.

Kodak Dental Radiography Series: Quality Control Tests for Dental Radiography. Kodak Health Sciences. Rochester, New York, Eastman Kodak Company, 1988.

Langland OE, Sippy FH, Langlais RP: Attenuation and recording the radiographic image. In Textbook of Dental Radiology, 2nd edition, p 88. Springfield, Illinois, Charles C Thomas, 1984.

Langland OE, Sippy FH, Langlais RP: X rays; their production, and the x-ray beam. In Textbook of Dental Radiology, 2nd edition, p 43. Springfield, Illinois, Charles C Thomas, 1984.

Mettler FA, Moseley RD: Basic radiation physics, chemistry, and biology. In Medical Effects of Ionizing Radiation, p 1. Orlando, Florida, Grune and Stratton, 1985.

Razmus TF: Radiation physics. In Miles DA, Van Dis ML, Razmus TF: Basic Principles of Oral and Maxillofacial Radiology, p 1. Philadelphia, WB Saunders, 1992.

Razmus TF, Glass BJ, McDavid WD: Comparison of image layer location among panoramic machines of the same manufacturer. Oral Surg Oral Med Oral Pathol 1989;67:102–108.

Richards AG: Radiation physics. In Goaz PW, White SC Oral Radiology: Principles and Interpretation, 3rd edition, p 1. St. Louis, CV Mosby, 1994.

3

CHARACTERISTICS OF IMAGE RECEPTORS AND PRODUCING DIAGNOSTIC QUALITY IMAGES

THOMAS F. RAZMUS

Overview of Image Receptors

X-Ray Film Composition

Intensifying Screens

Extraoral Film Cassettes

Film-Based Image Formation

Electronic Image Receptors

Image Receptors and Their Imaging Characteristics

Electronic Detector Structure and Mechanism of Image Capture

Quality of Digital Images

Digital Image Processing

Producing Diagnostic Quality Images

OVERVIEW OF IMAGE RECEPTORS

Chapter 3 discusses latent image formation in film-based systems and image acquisition in electronic imaging systems. Included in the discussion are direct exposure film, light-sensitive film and intensifying screens (film-screen combinations), electronic image receptors, and image display and manipulation.

Intraoral radiographic film is available in several sizes and speeds, and it is unique to dentistry. The most common sizes are designated as number 1 and number 2 periapical or bitewing film and occlusal film. The speed of a film refers to how sensitive the silver halide–containing emulsion is to radiation. Faster film is more sensitive to radiation and requires less exposure to make an image. The uniqueness of intraoral film lies in its mechanism of response to exposure by x rays.

Film used in dentistry to make extraoral images is the same as that employed in medicine to make the larger-format radiographs of the chest and extremities. Extraoral film (medical film) is available in several standard sizes, including 8 × 10 inches and 10 × 14 inches; larger sheets can be purchased. Panoramic machines require film that is 5 × 12 inches or 6 × 12 inches, depending on the brand of machine and the size of its film cassette. Extraoral films are designed to be used with intensifying screens.

Intraoral x-ray film and electronic image receptors are reacted upon by what remains of the primary radiation after it has passed through the patient. Such radiation is referred to as *remnant radiation*. The pattern projected by the remnant radiation will ultimately result in the radiographic or electronic image.

The way in which x-ray film responds to radiation results in two categories of film type: (1) *direct exposure,* or nonscreen, film, and (2) *light-sensitive,* or screen, film. Periapical, bitewing, and occlusal film react to direct exposure by x rays and are classified as direct exposure or nonscreen film. Panoramic and other extraoral radiographs are made with film that does not respond well to direct exposure by x rays but instead is designed to react to visible light; this is the *light-sensitive* or screen film. The light to which these films react is provided by an *intensifying screen.* Intensifying screens fluoresce (emit visible light) when exposed to x rays. Dyes are added to the emulsion of screen film to attract as much light from the fluorescing screen as possible. During an exposure, the screen film is held in intimate contact with the intensifying screen in a specialized case called a *cassette.*

Although the emulsion of screen film (light-sensitive film) contains essentially the same photosensitive silver halide as nonscreen film does, the added dyes, thinner emulsion layers, and decreased concentration of silver halide in screen film result in diminished photosensitivity to direct exposure by x radiation. Screen film must be used with a color-matched intensifying screen. Light-sensitive film and intensifying screens will be described later in this chapter.

Operators are cautioned that all x-ray film is sensitive to stray or scatter radiation and visible light and can be ruined by accidental exposure: proper handling and storage of film are essential.

X-RAY FILM COMPOSITION

The structural integrity and rigidity of x-ray film result from the *polyester,* plastic-like film base (Fig. 3–1). The base of extraoral films must provide enough stiffness to allow ease in handling larger format radiographs. Intraoral films, on the other hand, require enough flexibility to allow the corners to be gently folded or rolled when film placement is uncomfortable for the patient. Since images are viewed through the film base, there can be no irregularities in its composition. A blue tint added to the base makes details

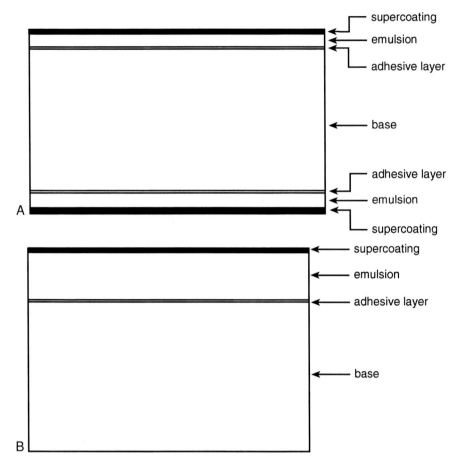

Figure 3–1. *A,* Components of a double emulsion film. *B,* Components of a single emulsion film.

easier to see and lessens eye fatigue. The base must also be able to withstand soaking in processing chemicals without degrading or distorting.

The *emulsion* is that part of the film where the visible radiographic image will eventually reside. The emulsion evenly covers both sides of the film base, although some films have emulsion on only one side. Double-emulsion films are faster (require less radiation to produce an image) and thus reduce radiation dose to the patient. Single-emulsion film provides increased image sharpness but has a higher exposure requirement. X-ray duplicating film is a specific type of single emulsion film. A very thin layer of adhesive holds the emulsion(s) to the base.

The emulsion has two principal components: photosensitive silver halide crystals and a gelatin that holds the crystals in suspension. The silver halide crystals, often referred to as *grains,* consist mostly (95%) of silver bromide and a lesser amount of silver iodide. The silver iodide and a very small quantity of a sulfur-containing crystal lattice contaminant increase the photosensitivity of the silver bromide crystals. The emulsion is coated with a protective layer of gelatin called the *supercoating.* The supercoating helps prevent scratching of the emulsion during film processing and handling. The supercoating and the gelatin making up the emulsion are porous, to allow the processing chemicals to react with the silver halide crystals.

An intraoral film base has an embossed *dot* located near one corner (Fig. 3–2). The dot is concave on one side and convex on the other and has several purposes. Radiographs to be taken by the paralleling technique and using a position-indicating device (PID) must have the edge of the film packet nearest the dot placed into the slot of the instrument's biteblock. This prevents the dot from potentially obscuring critical information on the processed radiograph. When a film is placed in the patient's mouth, the raised (convex) side of the dot must be toward the source of radiation. The dot is also used to determine the patient's left side films from right side films after they have been processed. The first step in the orientation of left and right side radiographs, prior to mounting, is accomplished by arranging the films on a flat surface such that the convex side of the dot is facing the operator.

Intraoral x-ray film is packaged in either a soft white plastic or paper wrapper. The packet wrapper is resistant to penetration by moisture such as saliva. When preparing to make a radiograph, the white side of the wrapper, which contains the convex side of the dot, is always positioned facing the source of radiation. The other side of the packet consists partially of colored paper that will correspond to a specific speed of film for that manufacturer. There may be one or two pieces of film within the packet, thus the designation of single-film packet or double-film packet. Double-film packets allow the clinician to place one film in the patient record and use the other film as a duplicate.

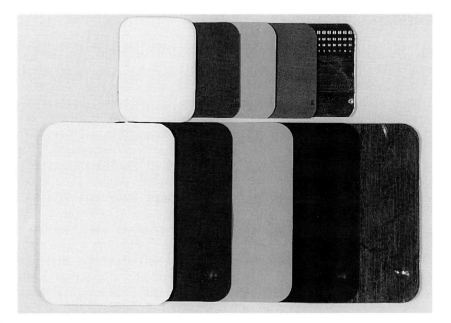

Figure 3–2. Intraoral film packets. The top packet is a number 2 size film used for adult periapical and/or bitewing radiography; the bottom packet is a number 4 size film used for occlusal projections. The components of each packet *(left to right)* are the white plastic wrapper, the first layer of black paper, the film, the second layer of black paper, and the lead foil. The white side of the plastic wrapper will always face the source of radiation during an exposure. An embossed dot is located in the lower right corner of each component.

Inside the wrapper the film is again wrapped, but this time with black paper. The black paper wrapper helps protect the film from exposure to light that may leak into the packet if it is handled roughly. A piece of lead foil corresponding in size to the film base is located between the black paper and external wrapper on the side of the packet away from the source of radiation. The lead foil helps prevent the film from becoming fogged by secondary radiation scattered back from the patient and may provide some reduction in radiation dose to the patient by attenuating the primary beam immediately after it has passed through the film base.

Dental radiographic films (intraoral and extraoral) use a double emulsion that may contain standard silver halide crystals or a modified form of the crystals. Standard crystals vary in size and shape throughout the emulsion. Modified crystals also vary in size but are described as (1) having a flat surface that allows more of the crystal to be exposed to radiation than the irregularly shaped conventional crystals, and (2) having the flat surfaces arranged in the emulsion so that they face the source of radiation. The flat grains are said to have a "tabular" shape and are used in Ektaspeed PLUS intraoral film and "T-Mat" extraoral film (Eastman Kodak Company, Rochester, New York). The benefit of the flat grains is to increase the speed of the film and reduce radiation dose without loss of image detail.

Dyes are added to the emulsion of screen film, and a specific *intensifying screen* and *film combination* must be used to assure that the wavelength of light produced by the intensifying screen will be compatible with the color of dye in the emulsion.

INTENSIFYING SCREENS

Intensifying screens are classified as *calcium tungstate* and *rare earth* screens. When exposed to x rays, intensifying screens emit visible light. Calcium tungstate screens will emit blue and blue-violet light and must be used only with *blue-sensitive* film. Standard silver halide films are *blue-sensitive,* and they will react to blue or blue-violet light. Exposure of rare earth screens to x rays causes them to emit green light. Film sensitive to green light must be matched to rare earth screens. Green-sensitive film is also called *orthochromatic,* or *ortho,* film. A mismatched film and intensifying screen combination will result in (1) greatly reduced speed of the film/screen system, (2) the need to retake the radiograph, and (3) increased dose to the patient resulting from the need to repeat the exposure. The reduced speed in this instance means that the film will not respond optimally to the light emitted by the incompatible screen. The resultant radiograph will be underexposed and too light to present reliable information about the patient. The appropriate film and intensifying screen combination will result in an image receptor system that is 10 to 60 times more sensitive to x rays than direct exposure film. Rare earth systems are approximately twice as fast as calcium tungstate systems.

As direct exposure film responds to the image pattern projected by remnant radiation exiting from the patient, intensifying screens perform this function in a light-sensitive film and intensifying screen system. Intensifying screens respond to radiation by emitting visible light through the process of *fluores-*

Table 3–1. Available Intensifying Screen/Light-Sensitive Film Combinations and Their Relative Speeds

Film and Screen Manufacturer	Screens/Color Emitted	Relative Speed of Compatible Films	
Kodak	Lanex/green light: Fine Medium Regular Fast	TMG and TML: 100 250 400 600	TMH: 250 600 800 1200
3 M	Trimax/green light: 2 4 8 12	XD/A and XL/A: 100 200 400 600	XM: 800 1200
Dupont	Quanta/blue light: Detail Fast detail Rapid	10T and 10TL: 100 200 400	

cence. The materials responsible for the fluorescence are called *phosphors.* The image seen on a processed light-sensitive film results from exposure of the film to the visible light emitted by the intensifying screen in proportion to the incident radiation. Tables 3–1 and 3–2 outline the features of several available light-sensitive films and intensifying screens.

Screen Composition

Intensifying screens consist of the base, the phosphor layer, the reflective layer, and a protective coating (Fig. 3–3).

Table 3–2. Imaging Characteristics of Light-Sensitive Films from Various Manufacturers

Manufacturer and Film	Imaging Characteristics
Kodak and T Mat G (TMG) 3 M and XD/A Dupont and 10T	Medium detail, medium speed, high contrast, narrow latitude
Kodak and T Mat L (TML) 3 M and XL/A Dupont and 10TL	Medium detail, medium speed, low contrast, wide latitude
Kodak and T Mat H (TMH) 3 M and XM	Low detail, high speed, high contrast, narrow latitude

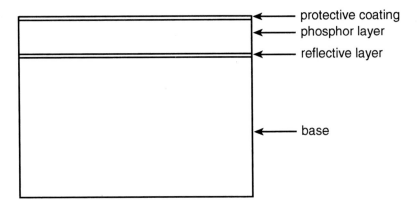

Figure 3–3. Components of an intensifying screen.

The *base* is the structural component upon which the other screen elements are applied. It is made of a polyester similar to the base of x-ray film and gives the screen its rigidity.

The *reflective layer* is a coating of white titanium dioxide applied to the base. The phosphor layer is applied over the reflective layer. The purpose of the reflective layer is to reflect stray light back to the x-ray film when the phosphor layer is exposed to x rays and emits light. This scavenging of stray light photons increases the efficiency and sensitivity of the screen system and contributes to dose reduction to the patient.

The *phosphor layer* contains the crystalline phosphor materials that fluoresce or emit visible light when exposed to x rays. The crystals are suspended in a plastic-like material that covers the reflective layer. As discussed earlier, screens emit a specific color of light depending on the type of phosphor present. Calcium tungstate crystals emit blue to blue-violet light, whereas crystals of rare earth elements emit light in the green range of the visible light spectrum.

Intensifying screens are so named because the phosphors convert one incident x-ray photon into many light photons, resulting in intensification or amplification of the response to a given photon energy. The light photons then expose the light-sensitive film. The outcome is that less radiation is used to produce a light-sensitive film image than that used to produce a direct exposure film image. Rare earth phosphors convert x-ray photons to light photons approximately two to four times more efficiently than calcium tungstate phosphors do. Imaging systems composed of green light–sensitive films and rare earth screens are the current state-of-the-art in film-based extraoral radiography.

A thin *protective coating* of flexible plastic covers the phosphor layer. The coating is durable enough to withstand repeated insertion and removal of film from the cassette while protecting the underlying phosphor layer. Screens must be cleaned regularly to prevent debris such as lint or paper from blocking the transmission of light to the film. When materials block light emitted from the screen and keep it from reaching the film, this will result in white (unexposed) or light (underexposed) areas on the processed film. Screens should be cleaned regularly and only with products specifically formulated for that purpose. These dedicated products not only clean the screen but also are antistatic agents that decrease the screen's attraction for dust and lint. Alcohol, dish-washing detergents, and other household cleaners should not be used on intensifying screens. Regular inspection of screens is necessary because cracks may occur after prolonged use or rough handling when inserting and removing film from the cassette. Screens placed in rigid cassettes are likely to outlast those in flexible cassettes.

EXTRAORAL FILM CASSETTES

Extraoral radiographs are made with the film enclosed in a cassette. Cassettes may be rigid or soft (Fig. 3–4). Both types of cassette are double-sided and open at one end by a hinge apparatus. An intensifying screen covers the internal surface of each side of the cassette, and a piece of light-sensitive film placed into the cassette will be tightly sandwiched between the two screens. Intimate screen-to-film contact is essential for obtaining a high-quality radiographic image. Cassettes need to be maintained to assure that they are light-tight and will provide proper screen-to-film contact.

FILM-BASED IMAGE FORMATION

Remnant radiation is what remains of the primary beam of x radiation after it has passed through the patient. Remnant radiation projects a pattern of radiation intensities that will ultimately result in the visible radiographic image, regardless of film type. When the remnant radiation acts upon direct exposure film, it activates silver atoms in the emulsion in a configuration dictated by the varying intensities within the beam. By comparison, the light-emitting phosphor in intensifying screens will be activated by the remnant radiation, and the resultant visible light, proportional to the pattern of radiation intensities in the beam, will expose the light-sensitive film. The exposure of either film type to the remnant radiation ultimately will result in activation of silver atoms in the emulsion and formation of an invisible image pattern. This invisible image is called the *latent image*. The latent image is converted into a *visible image* when the exposed film is processed.

Radiographic film processing has two major activities: *developing* and *fixing*. Developing causes the exposed, covalently bound silver atoms to precipitate in the emulsion as darkened neutral metallic silver atoms. The unexposed silver is dissolved and rinsed from the emulsion during the fixing and rinsing stages of processing.

The silver halide crystals in radiographic film emulsion are made of silver (Ag), iodine (I), and bromine (Br) atoms held together by their electrical forces, or valence charges. Binding of these atoms to form a crystal lattice results from a covalent relationship or sharing of loosely bound outer shell electrons among these atoms. The atoms exist as ions during the sharing of an electron (covalent bonding), i.e., neutral Ag atoms become positively charged Ag^+ ions, and neutral Br and I atoms become negatively charged Br^- and I^- ions. Ions are electrically charged and reactive, in contrast to atoms, which are electrically neutral and relatively stable. The surface of the

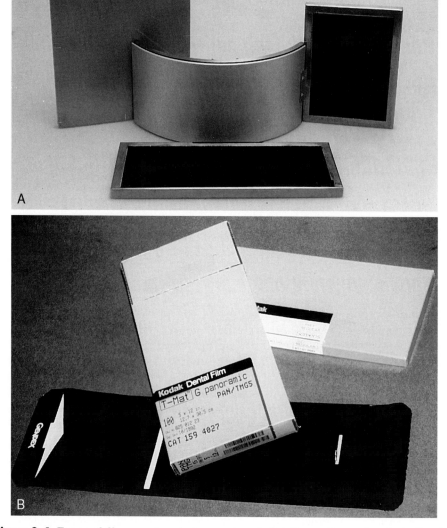

Figure 3–4. Extraoral film cassettes. *A,* An assortment of rigid cassettes made principally of steel. The curved and rectangular flat cassettes in the center of the picture are from different panoramic machines. *B,* An example of a flexible panoramic film cassette made of soft plastic.

silver halide crystal is negatively charged owing to the predominance of Br^- and I^- ions, whereas the center of the crystal contains most of the Ag^+ ions, resulting in an electrically balanced crystal structure. The surface of the crystal contains a defect in its lattice structure called a *sensitivity speck.* Film manufacturers commonly use sulfur-containing compounds such as *allylthiourea* to enhance formation of a sensitivity speck of silver sulfide. The purpose of the sensitivity speck is to capture electrons that have been freed from Br^- and I^- ions and create a negatively charged region on the crystal surface that will attract Ag$^+$ ions. These regions are called *latent image centers* and are where the latent image begins to form after exposure to x rays, or light from intensifying screens.

The *Gurney-Mott hypothesis* provides a general explanation of latent image formation. (1) Energy from an incident light or x-ray photon causes release (freeing) of an electron from Br$^-$ or I$^-$, resulting in formation of neutral Br or I. The Br or I is then released from the crystal into the gelatin. (2) The freed electron(s) is(are) attracted and held at the sensitivity speck. (3) The captured electron(s) attracts (attract) Ag$^+$ ion to the sensitivity speck, and the negative and positive charges cancel to form a neutral metallic Ag atom. (4) This first Ag atom attracts another Ag$^+$ ion by sharing an electron with the ion. Additional Ag$^+$ ions are attracted, neutralized, and bound into a mass of metallic silver atoms known as the latent image center. Processing chemicals, specifically the developing solution, act as a catalyst to continue precipitation of metallic Ag at latent image centers to form the visible image.

Manufacturers alter the formulations of their emulsions to vary and improve film characteristics such as speed, resolution, contrast, and latitude. These film characteristics will influence the radiographic technique selected and the features of resultant images. Modification of film characteristics is accomplished by varying the emulsion thickness; varying the concentration, shape, size, and orientation of silver halide crystals in the gelatin; and adding color-sensitive dyes to the emulsion.

ELECTRONIC IMAGE RECEPTORS

The electronic image receptor used for filmless or direct digital radiography creates its own version of a latent image. An electronic latent image is created when x rays activate electrons contained in the receptor. The electronic latent image is transferred to and stored in a computer and can be converted to a visible image on a video monitor or printed on paper.

There are two types of electronic image receptor designs: linear array and area array. Linear array detectors are generally used for extraoral projections such as skull radiography, tomography, and panoramic radiography, all of which involve scanning of a region of anatomy. Area array detectors are currently employed in a manner similar to intraoral periapical and bitewing film.

Two types of area array detectors exist: *fiberoptically coupled sensors* and *direct sensors.* That is to say, incident x rays interact with an intraorally positioned scintillation screen (intensifying screen) to produce visible light (photoelectrons) in proportion to the pattern projected by the remnant radiation. This is the same process (fluorescence) that occurs in a film-based intensifying screen system in which one x-ray photon interacting with the screen will generate many hundreds of light photons. In a fiberoptically coupled imaging system, the light is transmitted to the receptor via a lens system or fiberoptic device such as a flexible cable or rod. By comparison, direct exposure receptors are exposed to the remnant radiation and respond directly to the image pattern contained in the remnant beam, as does direct exposure film. Fiberoptically coupled systems have the receptors located remotely from the objects being imaged, whereas direct imaging systems employ an intraorally positioned detector. In both systems, the receptors store the latent image information as would a piece of film prior to processing. Chemical processing results in a visible film-based image; electronic or computer-based image processing results in a visible electronic image.

IMAGE RECEPTORS AND THEIR IMAGE CHARACTERISTICS

Both film-based and electronic images must possess certain visual properties to be considered of *diagnostic quality*. The physical principles governing each imaging modality result in technique-specific names being applied to analogous visual characteristics of an image, depending on whether it is film-based or electronic. The terminology in many cases is the same or similar, but, generally speaking, the theoretical basis is more complex when applied to electronic or computer-assisted imaging. Following are partial lists of terms commonly used to describe the characteristics of image receptors and images in film-based and electronic imaging.

Film-Based Imaging	*Electronic (Computer-Assisted)*
Radiographic density	*Imaging*
Radiographic contrast	Brightness
Film latitude	Contrast resolution
Film speed	Dynamic range
Radiographic mottle	Detector sensitivity
Image sharpness	Noise
Resolution	Spatial resolution

The remainder of this chapter discusses (1) the characteristics of radiographic film as an image receptor and how these characteristics affect film-based images, and (2) the characteristics of electronic image receptors or charge-coupled devices (CCDs) and how an electronic image is processed and manipulated. Throughout the discussion the characteristics of film-based images and electronic images will be related to one another when appropriate.

Film-based and electronic images must be of optimal *diagnostic quality* if they are to contribute accurate and dependable information to assist in making a diagnosis. Diagnostic quality requires that the image possess the proper *density* and adequate *contrast, sharpness,* and *resolution* for the diagnostic task at hand. A very significant point to remember is that an image without proper density cannot be relied upon to demonstrate optimal contrast, sharpness, or resolution (Fig. 3–5).

The film characteristics of base and fog density, overall density, contrast, speed, and latitude can be graphically displayed on a diagram called the *H & D (Hurter and Driffield) curve* or *characteristic curve.* Such a curve demonstrates the relationship of film exposure to density. Exposure results directly from the mAs, which determines the intensity of the x-ray beam or the number of x rays incident on the film—that is, intensity is directly proportional to density. Density is given on the vertical axis, and exposure is displayed horizontally (Fig. 3–6).

Recall that density is the overall darkness of the radiograph. Although density is described in terms of darkness and lightness of the radiograph, it is measured as the *amount of light transmitted* through the image. A density

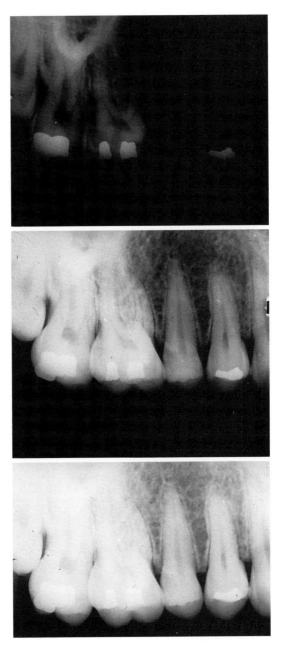

Figure 3–5. Three geometrically identical periapical projections. The difference among the images is the degree of density or overall darkness and the associated information yield. The middle image exhibits the most useful range of densities and presents the greatest amount of diagnostic information. The top image is too dark or dense to present any useful diagnostic information under standard viewing conditions. It may be possible to extract additional information from the dark image by viewing it in front of a high-intensity lamp called a "hot-light." The bottom image is too light in some areas to present complete information about the region covered by the film.

approaching zero means that nearly 100% of light is transmitted, or the radiograph is totally lucent except for the slight blue tint of the base. The range of useful radiographic densities is 0.5 (very light) to 2.5 (very dark). Outside these extremes the image is too light or too dark for diagnostic purposes, i.e., contrast, resolution, and sharpness within the image cannot be discerned (Fig. 3–7). Density is manipulated primarily by adjusting the exposure time, occasionally the mA, and to a lesser degree the kVp. Patient factors such as subject thickness and object density will affect density. A large

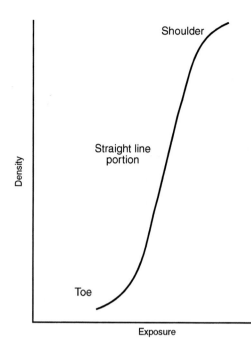

Figure 3–6. Characteristic curve or H & D curve named after Hurter and Driffield. The characteristic curve of a radiographic film is the graphic relationship between exposure and density. Large variations in exposure at both the lower (toe) and higher (shoulder) extremes of the curve will result in small changes in density. The straight-line or intermediate portion of the curve is where small variations in exposure will yield large changes in density. Radiographs with diagnostically useful densities will result when exposure factors in the straight-line portion of the curve are utilized.

Figure 3–7. Characteristic curve illustrating the various regions of the curve and the type of images produced in each region. Radiographs exhibiting a diagnostically useful range of densities between 0.5 and 2.5 will result from the straight-line portion of the curve. Excessively dark images will result from the shoulder region above density 2.5 and excessively light images from the toe region below density 0.5. Base and fog densities contribute no useful information to the image and should be kept as low as possible.

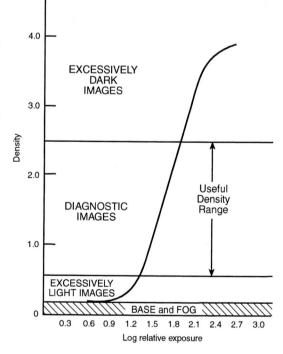

patient will most likely require a longer exposure time to maintain optimal density when compared with a smaller person. Occasionally a person may have unusually dense bone, in which case it may be necessary to increase the kVp to improve the penetrability of the x-ray beam.

Base and fog density contributes to the density or overall darkness of a radiograph. Base density results from the film base and the blue dye incorporated into the base. Fog density ideally should result only from the inadvertent exposure of a minimal amount of silver halide grains in the emulsion during manufacturing of the film. In reality, darkroom factors such as safe lighting and white light leaking into the darkroom, film freshness and storage conditions, and temperature and freshness of the processing solutions add to fog levels. The combination of base and fog is often indicated on an H & D curve as a horizontal line around density 0.2 (Fig. 3–7). Since fog results from random exposure of silver halide crystals in the emulsion, an unevenly distributed increase in the density of the radiograph further results in loss of the expected contrast and resolution. The lowest possible base and fog levels should be one of the goals of a radiology quality assurance (QA) program.

Contrast is defined as the difference in densities among the various regions of the image. Radiographic contrast is an analog characteristic, and therefore it is visible as continuous gradations from one shade of gray to another. A variable number of shades of gray exist in an image between the extremes of black and white. An image with many shades of gray between the extremes of black and white is said to have *low contrast,* or *long-scale contrast.* This degree of contrast is useful for detecting subtle changes in bone or soft tissue density. An image with few shades of gray between the extremes of black and white is said to have *high contrast,* or *short-scale contrast,* which is especially useful for the detection of interproximal caries. A high-contrast radiograph will appear more black and white overall when compared with a low-contrast radiograph, which would present as a softer image because of the more subdued appearance of the gray tones (see Fig. 1–1). An example of maximum high contrast or short-scale contrast is a black-and-white checkered flag. The relationship of contrast to x-ray beam attenuation was discussed in Chapter 2.

Factors that influence contrast are *kVp, subject contrast,* and *film contrast.* Kilovoltage peak is the exposure factor used to manipulate contrast. The maximum energy of the x-ray beam is determined by the kVp setting. A kVp such as 90 will generate a more energetic and, therefore, a more penetrating beam than a kVp of 75. The 90-kVp beam will penetrate varying densities within an object more uniformly and produce an image exhibiting subtle changes in density from one area to another, i.e., low contrast. A lower-energy beam generated at 75 kVp will be selectively absorbed to a greater degree as it travels through the same object. Different density or atomic number structures within the patient will have a greater effect on the lower-energy beam.

Subject contrast results from the thickness, density, and atomic number of the objects being imaged. The way in which subject contrast is displayed in an image is affected by kVp. An object of a given thickness, density, and atomic number will have a lesser effect on a higher-energy beam than on a lower-energy beam. Radiographing patients of different sizes, who may also possess different bone density, often necessitates adjusting the kVp setting in order to maintain or enhance contrast, depending on the diagnostic task. A simple rule can be applied when it becomes necessary to adjust the kVp:

Adjustment of the kVp must be of an adequate amount to effect an observable change in the image. Increments of 15 kVp are commonly used to increase or decrease contrast in the subsequent image. Recall that kVp also has an effect on density. A change of kVp calls for a corresponding change in one of the exposure factors that affect density. As discussed in Chapter 2, the most practical factor to manipulate to maintain the original density of the radiograph is the exposure time.

Film contrast is a function of how the emulsion is designed to react with incident x-ray or visible light photons. The reaction of the film depends on the characteristic (H & D) curve of the film, film processing, and the type of intensifying screen, if used.

The *slope,* or steepness, of the straight line portion of the characteristic (H & D) curve within the useful density range determines the inherent contrast of a film. The greater the slope (a steeper line), the greater the contrast (Fig. 3–8). It is desirable for a film to enhance subject contrast. Intraoral films will cause this to occur when the slope in the useful density range is greater than 1. The use of films with intensifying screens will increase the contrast to 2 or 3.

The contrast of a film is related to its latitude (Fig. 3–8). Film latitude refers to the range of exposure parameters that will produce images within the useful density range. A film with wide latitude can record objects that exhibit a broad range of subject contrast, i.e., the image will contain very dark regions, many shades of gray, and very light areas. Wide latitude films can portray a large proportion of the useful density range. The characteristic curve of a film with wide latitude will have a long straight line portion and a shallow (less steep) slope. Since wide latitude allows the demonstration of many shades of gray between the extremes of black and white, wide latitude

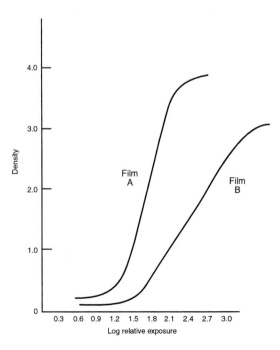

Figure 3–8. Characteristic curves exhibiting different contrast and latitude. The slope of the straight-line portion of Film A is steeper than that of Film B. Film A has greater contrast and narrower latitude than Film B.

films are selected when the diagnostic task calls for an image exhibiting low contrast. The characteristic curve of a narrow latitude film, on the other hand, will have a steeper slope and a more restricted range of useful exposure factor combinations. These films are selected for the higher contrast images that they produce. Latitude for electronic image receptors is referred to as *dynamic range*. The dynamic range for a CCD is extremely wide and much greater than the latitude of x-ray film. In addition to the inherent long-scale contrast offered by an electronic receptor, the image can also be subjected to computer manipulation to alter or enhance the contrast further.

Contrast varies with density to some extent and depends on where along the straight line portion of the characteristic curve the contrast is calculated. Since darker films have slightly more contrast than lighter films, contrast tends to increase as the shoulder of the characteristic curve is approached. This occurs because the darker elements of the image tend to overshadow the gray shades, resulting in an image that becomes predominantly black and white.

Film processing will affect radiographic contrast. Incomplete or excessive processing will result in loss of contrast. Deviation from the recommended processing time or temperature or using exhausted processing solutions will detract from contrast. Following the manufacturer's instructions for processing will yield optimal contrast from the film being used.

Contrast is negatively affected by *fog* and *scatter*. Fog is a nonuniform increase in the overall density of a radiograph; it carries no useful information and results in decreased contrast. As previously mentioned, fog results from accidental exposure to white light, unsafe safe-lighting conditions, film storage at high temperature, prolonged film development, or development at high temperatures. Scatter radiation from Compton scattering also results in an unevenly distributed increase in the overall darkness of the radiograph, increased fog levels, and loss of contrast. Excessive fog, regardless of its source, results in the loss of diagnostic information from the image. Using a kVp appropriate for the diagnostic task, collimating the beam to the size of the film or the area of interest, and using grids for extraoral techniques will reduce scatter radiation and fog.

Film speed refers to the sensitivity of film to radiation. By definition, speed is the amount of radiation needed to produce a density of 1.0 above base and fog (Fig. 3–9). A faster film will require less radiation to reach a particular density, and thus patient dose will be less. Intraoral film speed is designated by a letter such as D or E. The higher the letter designation, the faster the film. Light-sensitive film/intensifying screen combinations use numerical designations for the speed of the system, i.e., for a particular screen/film combination (see Table 3–1).

When characteristic curves are used to demonstrate the relative speed of two or more films, the curve for the faster film will be located to the left of the slower film, i.e., E-speed film will be to the left of D-speed film (Fig. 3–9).

Film speed is determined by the manufacturer. Closely guarded trade secrets are used to determine the size, shape, arrangement, and concentration of the silver halide grains in the emulsion, as well as the chemical composition of the emulsion itself. Since speed is designed into the film, a true alteration of the speed value is not possible. Attempts to increase speed indirectly by increasing development temperature will also result in increased fog and

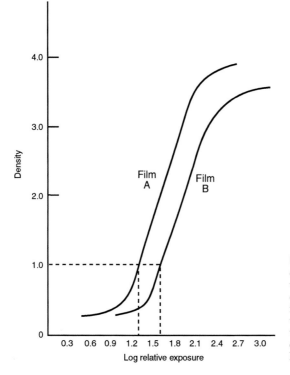

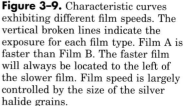

Figure 3–9. Characteristic curves exhibiting different film speeds. The vertical broken lines indicate the exposure for each film type. Film A is faster than Film B. The faster film will always be located to the left of the slower film. Film speed is largely controlled by the size of the silver halide grains.

graininess of the image. Electronic image receptors are much more sensitive to radiation than is x-ray film. The average CCD requires approximately 80% less exposure than E-speed film.

Sharpness is the ability of a radiograph to define the edge of an object. Sharpness is affected by machine factors, film factors, intensifying screen factors, and technique factors. Machine, film, and screen factors cannot be altered by the operator.

The size of the focal spot, determined by the manufacturer, affects image sharpness. A smaller focal spot will result in a sharper image. Focal spot size has a greater effect on image sharpness in film-based imaging than in electronic imaging. Sharpness in an electronic image cannot be manipulated by only using the computer, but additional factors that compose the electronic image must be accounted for, such as pixel size and the number of pixels in a given area, called spatial frequency.

In film-based imaging, the size of the Ag halide grains affects image sharpness. Smaller grains result in a sharper image, but also result in a slower film, longer exposure time, and higher patient dose. Generally, slower films have smaller grains, and faster films have larger grains. Processing at excessively high temperatures can result in the appearance of increased grain size, *film graininess,* and loss of sharpness.

Parallax is a type of image unsharpness that occurs with dental x-ray films because of their double emulsion configuration. Parallax results because the identical images in each emulsion are superimposed but separated by the thickness of the film base. The resulting unsharpness appears because the edges of the image in each emulsion can be seen.

Recall that intensifying screens expose light-sensitive film by emitting visible light when struck by x-ray photons. Light emitted from the screen diverges as it travels from its source to the film, which results in overlap of individual light beams. The divergent and overlapping beams of light expose an area of the film larger than their individual sources, which in turn results in blurring of the edges of objects. The inherent unsharpness of intensifying screen/film systems can be minimized by assuring intimate screen-to-film contact, thus reducing the distance the emitted light must travel from the screen to the film.

Screen speed affects image sharpness. The speed of a screen depends upon how efficiently it converts x-ray energy to light energy, which depends upon the composition and size of its phosphor crystals. Screen phosphors, as discussed earlier, are composed of calcium tungstate or rare earth elements. Larger phosphor crystals of either type will generate light more efficiently, resulting in a faster screen. A faster screen will reduce the patient dose but will result in loss of image sharpness—a situation analogous to film speed. Smaller phosphor crystals are less radiation sensitive, are less efficient at generating light, and require more exposure, but they result in a sharper image. A variety of films and screens are available to be matched in order to accomplish the diagnostic task being considered (see Tables 3–1 and 3–2).

Technique factors affecting image sharpness are (1) motion of the object or x-ray source during the exposure, (2) source-to-film distance, and (3) object-to-film distance. Motion unsharpness can be minimized by using the shortest practical exposure time. Image projection factors such as source-to-film distance and object-to-film distance contribute to geometric unsharpness. Geometric unsharpness can be minimized by using the longest practical source-to-film distance and the shortest possible object-to-film distance. The shape and thickness of the object will also influence image sharpness. These relationships are discussed thoroughly in the section dealing with the production of diagnostic quality images.

Resolution is the ability of a radiograph to record and demonstrate separate objects that are close together. Resolution can be measured by using a test device that contains several lead strips embedded in an acrylic wafer (Fig. 3–10). The lead strips become progressively narrower as the wafer is observed from one end to the other. The basis of this test procedure is that a greater number of narrower strips can fit into a like amount of space, 1 millimeter. The unit of measurement is referred to as a line pair and consists of one lead strip and an adjacent radiolucent space of acrylic. Resolving power is thus measured in line pairs per millimeter (lp per mm). Periapical films resolve from 10 to 16 lp per mm, panoramic and other light-sensitive film/intensifying screen combinations up to about 5 lp per mm, and a typical CCD up to approximately 10 lp per mm. The human eye can detect in the area of 4 to 6 lp per mm. Resolution, like sharpness, is affected by focal spot size, motion, and properties of the image receptor.

Intraoral direct digital imaging employs the same type of x-ray machine as is used to create a film-based image; consequently, focal spot size, motion, and geometric factors will also influence digital image sharpness and resolution. The CCDs used for intraoral imaging are area array, two-dimensional detectors that produce an image by direct projection, as in film-based intraoral imaging. Linear array detectors, as used to acquire larger format images such

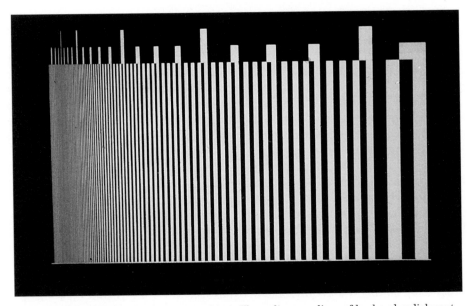

Figure 3–10. A line-pair resolution test object. The radiopaque lines of lead and radiolucent spaces of acrylic become narrower and more closely spaced from one end of the device to the other. (Courtesy of Dr. Robert G. Pifer, West Virginia University School of Dentistry, Morgantown, West Virginia.)

as extraoral projections, require a scanning motion of the x-ray beam to create an image. Characteristic image artifacts result from the motion factor accompanying image capture by a linear array detector. An image from an area array detector will exhibit higher levels of sharpness and resolution than one acquired by a linear detector. Since both the intraoral area array detector and the extraoral linear detector are linked to a computer, a certain degree of manipulation of image sharpness and resolution is possible in either case.

ELECTRONIC DETECTOR STRUCTURE AND MECHANISM OF IMAGE CAPTURE

The production of film-based images results from a chemical reaction initiated when light from the intensifying screens or the x-ray energy in the remnant beam interacts with the silver halide crystals in the film emulsion. Electronic images result when light from the system's image receptor or x-ray energy in the remnant beam is converted into electrical energy in the CCD. Electronic images are mathematical models of the energy intensities contained in the remnant beam. These mathematical models are called *algorithms*. Algorithms allow an image to be manipulated through mathematical operations performed by the computer.

Most CCDs are made from pure silicon (Fig. 3–11). The electrons in the wafer of silicon comprising a CCD can be visualized as being subdivided into a pixel arrangement. Each pixel is referred to as an *electron potential well*. X-ray photons incident on the CCD will cause electrons to be released from

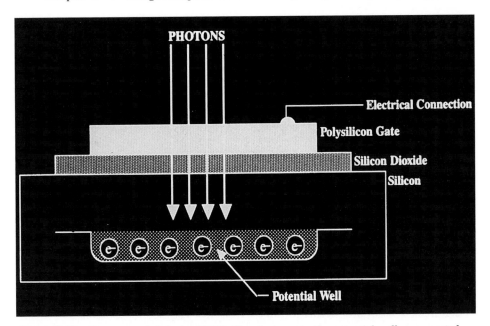

Figure 3-11. Charge-coupled device (CCD). The electrons in the potential wells are reacted upon by x-ray photons in the remnant beam of radiation to create an electronic latent image. (Courtesy of Dr. S. Brent Dove, University of Texas Dental School at San Antonio, Texas.)

the silicon. Since preexposed silicon electrons are subdivided into the electron well configuration, electrons freed by exposure to remnant radiation will remain in their respective wells. The number of electrons released by a photon interaction is, therefore, quantified for each well. An electric charge proportional to the energy of the incident radiation will be generated when electrons are released; consequently, each pixel (electron potential well) will contain an electric charge proportional to the energy of the incident photons and the number of electrons reacted with in the well.

The total charge in each electron potential well is transferred to an output amplifier that increases the relatively weak voltage into a measurable signal. These signals constitute an analog (continuous gray tone) video image. An analog-to-digital converter measures the voltage at specific intervals throughout the analog image and assigns a number proportional to the intensity of charge at each site measured. Each number corresponds to a specific shade of gray and is the digital equivalent of the analog image. Data are stored in the computer memory component called a *frame grabber.*

QUALITY OF DIGITAL IMAGES

Film-based images must possess the appropriate density for image contrast, sharpness, and resolution to be optimal. Electronic images depend upon the digital image features of *contrast resolution* and *spatial resolution* to produce optimal image quality.

Regardless of whether the digital image was obtained with an area array detector or by digitization of a radiograph, the original image will have been in analog format and subsequently converted to the digital configuration. *Contrast resolution* is a measure of how accurately the digital image pixel brightness compares with the brightness (density) at the same location in the original (analog) image. In a very general way, digital image brightness is comparable to the density of a film-based or analog image. Contrast resolution will affect contrast within the digital image. The accuracy of the digital image pixel brightness depends on the number of shades of gray in the gray scale produced by the image-processing equipment. The accepted standard of accuracy is 256 levels (shades) of gray, or an 8-bit image.

Spatial resolution of a digital image is a measure of the extent to which the displayed digital image appears identical to the original (analog) image. Spatial resolution is determined by the number and size of the pixels used to compose the displayed digital image. The higher the number and the smaller the pixel size used to portray the original image, the closer its appearance will be to the original image. Spatial resolution affects image contrast and sharpness. Maximal spatial resolution, which would result in the most accurate representation of the original (analog) image and its inherent changes in brightness from one detail to another, would require more than 256 levels of gray. Such a degree of image processing would require digitizing or forming pixels (analog-to-digital conversion) at a rate at least twice as great as the highest rate of brightness (density) change within the original analog image. The hardware that determines spatial resolution is the frame grabber, and most of this hardware provides for a spatial resolution of 512 pixels $\times$ 512 pixels or 640 pixels $\times$ 480 pixels. These two numbers describe the size of the image matrix as the number of pixels in the lines and columns composing the digital image. The amount of computer memory needed to store or transmit an image is greatly affected by the level of contrast and spatial resolution. Higher resolution frame grabbers are available, but they are too costly to be practical for dental applications.

DIGITAL IMAGE PROCESSING

Image processing includes those procedures that allow visual enhancement or quantitative assessment of some aspect of the displayed digital image not discernible from the original (analog) image. Image processing was used extensively by NASA in the 1960s to study the moon's surface in preparation for the Apollo space program. Images to be processed possess three properties: (1) contrast, or the difference in brightness between two regions of the image, (2) spatial frequency, which is a measure of the rate of change of brightness from one point in the image to another, and (3) noise, which is any distracting information in the image, i.e., information that does not contribute to the diagnostic usefulness of the image.

Image processing consists of three basic operations: *analysis operations, enhancement operations,* and *encoding operations.*

Analysis operations result in numerical information that describes some aspect of the image not visually apparent, e.g., how many pixels have a certain gray value. Image histograms, which resemble a bar graph, can be constructed to illustrate the distribution of gray levels among the pixels composing an image. An analysis of density or brightness can be used to demonstrate the intensity or gray value at a specific point in an image, e.g., to assess changes in bone density over time. Digital formatting facilitates the dimensional analyses of the length, width, spatial orientation, circumference, or area occupied by structures in the image. These analysis operations can provide information that may increase the diagnostic yield from an image.

Enhancement operations are used to modify the appearance of an image and improve the perceptibility of some feature within the image. Computer-based imaging in dentistry applies enhancement methods most commonly (1) to manipulate adjacent gray values to alter image contrast; (2) to intensify or subdue selected spatial frequencies within an image by attenuating or eliminating selected noise from the image (spatial frequencies are attenuated by high, median, or low pass spatial filtration); (3) to remove the structured noise of normal radiographic detail to make variations from normal or true pathosis more easily seen by the human observer, called digital subtraction radiography; and (4) to add pseudocolor to images.

Since the human eye can discern only 28 to 32 shades of gray as compared with the thousands of shades of different colors, it would seem that color enhancement would be a very beneficial manipulation. This would be true if the colors given to the components of an image actually meant the same thing each time. The problem is that colors are randomly assigned when used for enhancement purposes, and there is no standardized color scale upon which to base consistent judgments.

Encoding operations are applied when it is beneficial to reduce the information in an image to include only what is essential to describe the object accurately. Elimination of extraneous information allows more diagnostically significant information to be stored in a given amount of computer memory, or it allows more critical image information to be transmitted in a given transmission time. The two ways in which images can be encoded are *lossless algorithms* and *lossy algorithms*.

Lossless algorithms allow encoded information to be used to reconstruct an image that is identical to the original image. Lossless algorithms are mathematical models that result in no loss of image information, but they require more computer memory to perform the manipulations and more transmission time to transfer the image to another site.

Lossy algorithms result in the loss of some nonessential information from the original image. Although some information is lost, less computer memory is needed to perform the operations, and the data can be transmitted in a shorter period of time. Encoding in this manner can be used for *image compression* to facilitate storage and transmission of image data. Whether lossless or lossy encoding is applied to a specific set of images depends upon the task for which the encoded image(s) will be used to accomplish.

PRODUCING DIAGNOSTIC QUALITY IMAGES

A *diagnostic quality* image will exhibit a density that allows the other visual features of the image to be discernible. Optimal density will allow assessment of the image for the expected contrast, sharpness, and resolution. All these visual features will be compromised if the image is excessively dark or light. The manipulation of density and contrast has been discussed earlier in association with the x-ray machine controls affecting these image features and in relation to the various image receptors and their imaging characteristics. By this time the reader should have an understanding of how to select the appropriate exposure factor combination and image receptor to produce an image with optimal density and contrast for the diagnostic task being contemplated.

In addition to possessing optimal density and contrast, certain *geometric characteristics* of an image must be controlled and minimized to produce an accurate representation of the object being imaged. The three geometric features of the image are *unsharpness, magnification,* and *distortion.* Certain principles of image formation make it impossible to totally eliminate unsharpness, magnification, and distortion from images. These principles involve the size of the x-ray source, the divergence of the x-ray beam as it travels from its source, and the three-dimensional nature of the objects being imaged.

Image Unsharpness

Image unsharpness is the fuzziness surrounding the borders or edges of objects in an image. There are three types of image unsharpness: *geometric, motion,* and *screen* unsharpness.

GEOMETRIC UNSHARPNESS

Geometric unsharpness is influenced by the size of the x-ray source, the source-to-object distance, and the object-to-image-receptor distance. If the x rays used to produce diagnostic images were to originate from a single, infinitely small point source, the unsharpness due to this factor would be eliminated. Recall that x rays are generated over an area of the tungsten target called the focal spot. This area will vary from 0.5 to 1.5 mm^2. When individual electrons from the heated cathode filament make an impact on the focal spot, each point of impact acts as a point source for x-ray production. This results in a variable number of x-ray point sources in close proximity to one another. The outcome is that a variable number of individual x-ray beams will pass through the object and strike the image receptor at an equally variable number of different angles. The image created by this process will actually have a number of edge outlines. The eye combines these edges into what appears to be an unsharpness, or edge gradient (penumbra), surrounding the image. A greater source-to-object distance and a lesser object-to-receptor distance will result in less geometric unsharpness or penumbra (Fig. 3–12).

MOTION UNSHARPNESS

Motion unsharpness results from movement of any one or combination of the patient, the film, or the x-ray source during the exposure. Motion of the

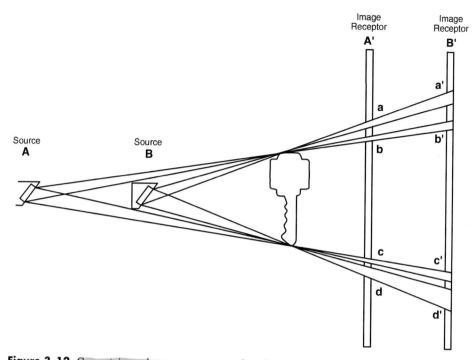

Figure 3–12. Geometric unsharpness, or penumbra. Images will exhibit the blurring of geometric unsharpness or penumbra when the x-ray source is a measurable area rather than an infinitely small point source. **Penumbra will be small when the object-to-image receptor distance (OID) is small.** X rays originating at either source A or B will result in a smaller penumbra at image receptor A′ (a, b, c, d) than at image receptor B′ (a′, b′, c′, d′). **Penumbra will be small when the source-to-object distance (SOD) is great.** Penumbra resulting from x rays originating at source A will be less at image receptor A′ (b, b′) and B′ (c, c′) than from x rays from source B (a, a′ and d, d′). **Image magnification is affected by SOD and OID.** Magnification resulting from x rays originating at source A will be less at image receptor A′ and B′ than from x rays originating at source B.

film or patient during the exposure is likely to cause the greatest degree of image unsharpness (Fig. 3–13). Vibration of the tubehead during an intraoral film exposure will result in an enlarged focal spot and contribute to an increase in image unsharpness.

SCREEN UNSHARPNESS

As discussed earlier, intensifying screens emit visible light to expose a compatible light-sensitive film in extraoral radiographic procedures. The phosphor layer contains the fluorescing elements that are the light source of intensifying screens. Each x-ray photon interacting with the phosphor layer creates a point source for many photons of visible light, in essence creating a divergent beam of light that will expose the light-sensitive film. Since the point sources of light in the phosphor layer are closely approximated to one another, the divergent beams of light will overlap, and adjacent areas of the film will be exposed by the overlapping light beams. This is referred to as the

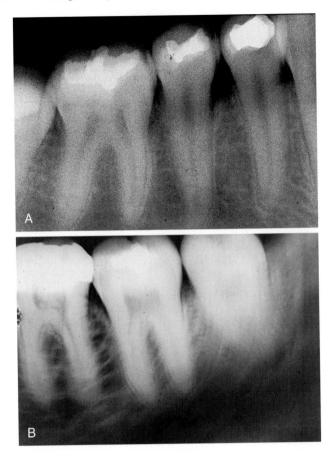

Figure 3–13. Motion unsharpness of teeth and adjacent bone. *A,* Slight motion unsharpness. *B,* Significant motion unsharpness (*B,* courtesy of Dr. Robert G. Pifer, West Virginia University School of Dentistry, Morgantown, West Virginia.)

cross-over effect and results in unsharpness of the resultant image. Intimate screen-to-film contact in the cassette will help minimize such unsharpness. Another factor contributing to screen unsharpness is the size of the crystals in the phosphor layer, which is related to the speed of the screen.

Magnification

Magnification is the equal enlargement of the object in the image. Factors that affect magnification are the same as those that influence geometric unsharpness, but the focal spot size plays a minor role.

The divergent behavior of the beam, even if it is a single beam originating from an infinitely small point source, will result in magnification of the object. Since a typical x-ray beam originates from an area (focal spot) rather than a point source, the image produced will always demonstrate some degree of magnification as well as geometric unsharpness.

Manipulation of the source-to-object and object-to-receptor distances can

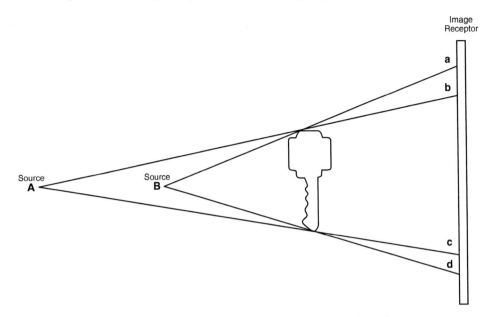

Figure 3–14. Magnification. An infinitely small x-ray point source will result in image magnification without geometric unsharpness.

have a notable effect on magnification. Magnification of dental structures can be minimized by increasing the source-to-object distance and reducing the object-to-receptor distance as far as practical (Fig. 3–14).

Distortion

Distortion is a variation of the true shape of the object resulting from unequal magnification or enlargement of parts of the object in the image. Creating images with x rays and an image receptor entails the recording of three-dimensional objects in a two-dimensional medium. Principles of image formation result in objects being located closest to the image receptor exhibiting the least amount of unsharpness, magnification, and distortion. When considering the entire depth of the three-dimensional object, unequal magnification of different parts of the object will occur because the various parts are located at different distances from and in different relationships to the image receptor. Distortion can be minimized by aligning the object, film, and the primary beam of radiation (Fig. 3–15). The principles of accurate image formation are discussed in Chapter 5.

In summary, a diagnostic quality image is created by the proper interaction of the following factors:

- **X-ray machine factors**
  Focal spot size (not adjustable; determined by the manufacturer)
    Affects geometric unsharpness and magnification
  Kilovoltage (kVp control setting)
    Regulates the penetration characteristics of the beam

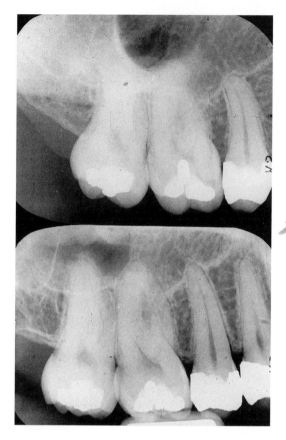

Figure 3–15. Image distortion. Because dental structures are composed of different three-dimensional configurations located at different angles and distances from the image receptor, unequal magnification or distortion of these components will appear in the image. Lingual cusps of teeth lie closest to the image receptor and will be imaged the sharpest and with the least distortion. Buccal cusps will be slightly magnified and may be elongated or foreshortened and imaged in a slightly different vertical plane than lingual cusps.

Regulates the contrast of the image
Affects the density of the image
Affects fog from scatter radiation
Affects exposure latitude
Affects patient dose
Milliampere-seconds (mAs)—mA control setting and/or exposure timer setting
Regulates the density of the image

- **Operator technique/geometrical factors**
Source-to-film and object-to-receptor distances
Affect image density, unsharpness, and magnification
Alignment of the film, object, and primary beam
Affects anatomical accuracy of the image, distortion, and anatomical coverage

REFERENCES

Brooks SL, Miles DA: Advances in diagnostic imaging in dentistry. Dento Maxillofac Radiol 1993;37(1):91–111.
Bushong SC: The atom. In Radiologic Science for Technologists: Physics, Biology, and Protection, 4th edition, p 30. St. Louis, CV Mosby, 1988.

Bushong SC: X-ray emission. In Radiologic Science for Technologists: Physics, Biology, and Protection, 4th edition, p 173. St. Louis, CV Mosby, 1988.

Bushong SC: Beam-restricting devices. In Radiologic Science for Technologists: Physics, Biology, and Protection, 4th edition, p 182. St. Louis, CV Mosby, 1988.

Bushong SC: Radiographic film. In Radiologic Science for Technologists: Physics, Biology, and Protection, 4th edition, p 212. St. Louis, CV Mosby, 1988.

Bushong SC: Processing the latent image. In Radiologic Science for Technologists: Physics, Biology, and Protection, 4th edition, p 225. St. Louis, CV Mosby, 1988.

Bushong SC: Intensifying screens. In Radiologic Science for Technologists: Physics, Biology, and Protection, 4th edition, p 241. St. Louis, CV Mosby, 1988.

Bushong SC: Radiographic quality. In Radiologic Science for Technologists: Physics, Biology, and Protection, 4th edition, p 258. St. Louis, CV Mosby, 1988.

Bushong SC: Radiographic technique. In Radiologic Science for Technologists: Physics, Biology, and Protection, 4th edition, p 290. St. Louis, CV Mosby, 1988.

Bushong SC: Digital x-ray imaging. In Radiologic Science for Technologists: Physics, Biology, and Protection, 4th edition, p 363. St. Louis, CV Mosby, 1988.

Conover GL, Hildebolt CF, Anthony D: Objective and subjective evaluations of Kodak Ektaspeed Plus dental x-ray film. Oral Surg Oral Med Oral Pathol 1995;79(2):246–250.

Cook LT, Giger ML, Wetzel LH, et al: Digitized film radiography. Invest Radiol 1989;24:910–916.

Dagenais ME, Clark BG: Receiver operating characteristics of RadioVisioGraphy. Oral Surg Oral Med Oral Pathol 1995;79(2):238–245.

Dove SB: Digital imaging in dentistry. American Academy of Oral and Maxillofacial Radiology NEWSLETTER, Winter 1992;19(1).

Dove SB, McDavid WD: A comparison of conventional intra-oral radiography and computer imaging techniques for the detection of proximal surface dental caries. Dento Maxillofac Radiol 1992;21(3):127–134.

Dove SB, McDavid WD: Digital panoramic and extraoral imaging. Dent Clin North Am 1993;37(4):541–551.

Goaz PW, White SC: X-ray film, intensifying screens, and grids. In Oral Radiology: Principles and interpretation, 3rd edition, p 79. St. Louis, CV Mosby, 1994.

Goaz PW, White SC: Projection geometry In Oral Radiology: Principles and Interpretation, 3rd edition, p 97. St. Louis, CV Mosby, 1994.

Grondahl HG, Grondahl K: Subtraction radiography for the diagnosis of periodontal bone lesions. Oral Surg Oral Med Oral Pathol 1983;55:208–213.

Grondahl HG, Grondahl K, Webber RL: Influence of variation in projection geometry on the detectability of periodontal bone lesions. A comparison between subtraction radiography and conventional radiographic technique. J Clin Periodontol 1984;11:411–420.

Horner K, Shearer AC, Walker A, et al: RadioVisioGraphy: An initial evaluation. Br Dent J 1990;168:244–248.

Kundel HL, Revesz G: Lesion conspicuity, structured noise and film reader error. Am J Roentgenol 1976;126:1233–1238.

Langland OE, Sippy FH, Langlais RP: Attenuation and recording the radiographic image. In Textbook of Dental Radiology, 2nd edition, p 88. Springfield, Illinois, Charles C Thomas, 1984.

Langland OE, Sippy FH, Langlais RP: Diagnostic quality of dental radiographs. In Textbook of Dental Radiology, 2nd edition, p 130. Springfield, Illinois, Charles C Thomas, 1984.

Ludlow JB, Platin E: Densitometric comparisons of Ultra-speed, Ektaspeed, and Ektaspeed Plus intraoral films for two processing conditions. Oral Surg Oral Med Oral Pathol 1995;79(1):105–113.

McDavid WD, Dove SB, Welander U, et al: Direct digital extraoral radiography of the head and neck with a solid-state linear x-ray detector. Oral Surg Oral Med Oral Pathol 1992;74:811–817.

McMillan JH, Huang HKB, Bramble JM, et al: Digital radiography. Invest Radiol 1989;24:735–741.

Miles, DA: Imaging using solid-state detectors. Dent Clin North Am 1993;37(4):531–540.

Miles DA, Van Dis ML, Razmus TF: Radiographic image production and film characteristics. In Basic Principles of Oral and Maxillofacial Radiology, p 49. Philadelphia, WB Saunders, 1992.

Mouyen R, Benz C, Sonnabend, et al: Presentation and physical evaluation of Radio-VisioGraphy. Oral Surg Oral Med Oral Pathol 1989;68:238–242.

Nelvig P, Wing K, Welander U: Sens-A-Ray: A new system for direct digital intraoral radiography. Oral Surg Oral Med Oral Pathol 1992;74:818–823.

Ohki M, Okano T, Nakamura T: Factors determining the diagnostic accuracy of digitized conventional intraoral radiographs. Dento Maxillofac Radiol 1994; 23(2):77–82.

Razzano MR, Bonner PJ: RadioVisioGraphy; Video imaging alters traditional approach to radiography. Compend Contin Educ Dent 1990;11(6):398–400.

Reddy MS, Jeffcoat MK: Digital subtraction radiography. Dent Clin North Am 1993;37(4):553–565.

Rethman M, Ruttiman V, O'Neal R, et al: Diagnosis of bone lesions by subtraction radiography. J Clin Periodontol 1985;56:324–329.

Revesz G, Kundel HL, Graber MA: The influence of structured noise on the detection of radiologic abnormalities. Invest Radiol 1974;9:479–486.

Thunthy KH, Weinberg R: Sensitometric comparisons of dental films of group D and E. Oral Surg Oral Med Oral Pathol 1982;54:250–252.

Thunthy KH, Weinberg R: Sensitometric comparison of Kodak Ektaspeed Plus, Ektaspeed, and Ultraspeed dental films. Oral Surg Oral Med Oral Pathol 1995;79(1):114–116.

Thunthy KH, Weinberg R: Effects of developer exhaustion on Kodak Ektaspeed Plus, Ektaspeed, and Ultraspeed dental films. Oral Surg Oral Med Oral Pathol 1995;79(1):117–121.

Tyndall DA, Kapa SF, Bagnell CP: Digital subtraction radiography for detecting cortical and cancellous bone changes in the periapical region. J Endodont 1990;16:173–178.

vander Stelt PF: Practical digital imaging; The future role of digital imaging in dentistry and in oral and maxillofacial radiology. American Academy of Oral and Maxillofacial Radiology NEWSLETTER, Winter 1994;21(1).

Zubery Y: Computerized image analysis in dentistry: Present status and future applications. Compend Contin Educ Dent 1993;8(11):964–973.

4

THE BIOLOGICAL EFFECTS AND SAFE USE OF RADIATION

THOMAS F. RAZMUS

Concepts of Radiation Exposure, Dose, and Measurement

Sources of Radiation Exposure

Occupational and Nonoccupational Radiation Exposure

Exposure and Dose from Oral and Maxillofacial Diagnostic Imaging

Risk from Dental Diagnostic Radiography

Effects of Ionizing Radiation on Living Systems

Methods to Reduce Exposure and Dose from Dental Diagnostic Radiography

Risk from Diagnostic Imaging with Nonionizing Radiation

Design Features of a Radiation-Safe Dental Facility

Hazardous Waste in Radiography

Radiation can be either *ionizing* or *nonionizing*. X rays are a form of ionizing radiation because they create positive and negative ions by inter-acting with the orbital electrons of atoms. Other forms of ionizing radiation, called particulate radiation, also ionize matter but with greater frequency and intensity than x rays. The diagnostic techniques of *ultrasound* and *magnetic resonance imaging* employ nonionizing forms of radiation to create diagnostic images. Although no harmful effects have been demonstrated from the use of these two imaging modalities to diagnose conditions in humans, the benefits should always outweigh the risks in their application.

Radiation biology is the study of the effects of ionizing radiation on biologi-cal tissue. The measures taken to assure that radiation workers and the general population receive the absolute minimal dose of radiation when performing a specific task are referred to as *radiation protection* measures. Radiation protection practices are based on the findings of radiobiological research. Research data have come from studies of various populations that were exposed to doses of radiation much higher than those used in diagnostic imaging. The exposure of these populations was the result of war, accident, occupation, or medical treatment deemed correct at the time.

Since diagnostic imaging employs relatively low doses of radiation with no observable negative effects, it was necessary to extrapolate the risk data from these highly exposed groups in order to apply it to potential damage from low-dose, low-intensity exposure. The pervasive message in *radiation safety doctrine* is that *no dose of radiation is a safe dose.* The guiding principle is that the dose of radiation used to create a diagnostic image must be "As Low As Reasonably Achievable," or the *"ALARA principle."*

CONCEPTS OF RADIATION EXPOSURE, DOSE, AND MEASUREMENT

A discussion of the biological effects of radiation includes constant reference to radiation exposure and dose levels. The units of radiation measurement must be at least familiar to the reader for such a discussion to be meaningful.

Two systems of nomenclature are applied to the units of radiation measurement: the Standard System and the SI or Système Internationale (International System). The Standard System has been used most commonly in this country and includes the units of the *roentgen (R), rad,* and *rem.* The SI was most recently adopted by the international scientific community and will eventually replace the roentgen (R) with the coulomb* per kilogram *(C/kg),* the rad with the *gray* (Gy), and the rem with the *sievert* (Sv).

The roentgen was named for Wilhelm Konrad Roentgen, discoverer of the x ray. The roentgen or coulomb per kilogram is the unit of exposure and refers to the ability of x rays to ionize air. When a determination of patient exposure is to be made, the measurement is taken at the skin surface and before the radiation has penetrated the patient. This unit is used only to determine exposure to x rays or gamma rays. By definition, it is the quantity of radiation capable of ionizing 1.6×10^{12} ion pairs per gram of air. An exposure of 1.0 R is equal to an electric charge of 2.58×10^{-4} C/kg of air, or approximately 87 ergs† per gram of air. Instruments used to measure radiation exposure will display machine output in roentgens (R) or milliroentgens (mR), or C/kg, or both.

The rad (radiation absorbed dose) is the unit of absorbed dose and is most often used when describing the quantity of radiation dose received by a patient or other biological system. It quantifies the amount of ionizing radiation energy absorbed per gram of tissue. An exposure of water or soft tissue by 1.0 R of x rays or gamma rays results in an absorbed dose of 1.0 rad; note

---

*Coulomb (C): A unit of quantity of electricity; the amount of electricity provided by a current of 1.0 ampere in 1.0 second.
†erg: The unit of work in the centimeter/gram/second (CGS) system.

that this 1:1 relationship applies only to these two types of radiation. The gray (Gy) is equivalent to 100 rad. Very small absorbed doses are measured in millirad (mrad) or milligray (mGy). The following relationships should be familiar to radiation operators.

Relationships of Exposure to Absorbed Dose

1.0 R = 0.87 rad = 87 ergs/g of air

1.0 rad = 0.01 Gy = 0.01 J*/kg

1.0 Gy = 100 rad = 1.0 J/kg = 114 R

The many different forms of ionizing radiation will transfer their inherent energy to biological organisms at different rates and in varying degrees of intensity; consequently, different types of radiation will affect living systems in different ways. Particulate radiations (alpha particles or protons) will transfer energy to biological tissues much more rapidly and intensely than electromagnetic radiations (x rays). Particulate radiations are much more damaging to living systems than x rays or gamma rays. To account for the variability of the biological effectiveness per unit of absorbed dose for each different type of ionizing radiation, the *quality factor* (QF) and *relative biological effectiveness* (RBE) were developed. Biological effectiveness refers to the efficiency with which a certain type of radiation will produce a given effect.

The RBE is a radiobiological concept used to compare the biological effectiveness of any type of radiation to a standard or test radiation in producing the same biological effect or biological end-point, e.g., erythema, cancer, cataracts. The QF is a value assigned to each of the several types of radiation to rank them according to their RBE. The QF value is used as a multiplier with absorbed dose to calculate the *dose equivalent* (DE) for radiation protection purposes.

The dose equivalent (DE) is a calculated value that expresses on a common scale the biological damage an exposed individual might expect to incur from a particular type of radiation. Experimental data have shown that an absorbed dose of one type of radiation will not produce the same biological effect as the same dose of another type of radiation. The DE is used to compare the risk of a biological effect from specified doses of different types of radiation. The DE is the product of the absorbed dose and quality factor. The rem (radiobiological equivalent man) or sievert (Sv) is the unit used to express dose equivalent.

DE = rad or gray × QF

When the absorbed dose is expressed in gray, dose equivalent will be expressed in sieverts; absorbed dose expressed in rads necessitates that dose equivalent be in rems. Recall that the quality factor is only a ranking multiplier and has no units.

Occupational exposure of radiation workers is monitored in the dose equivalent unit of rem or Sv, usually as millirem (mrem) or millisievert (mSv)

---

*joule (J): The unit of work in the meter/kilogram/second (MKS) system.

because the dose being monitored is quite small. Since some types of ionizing radiation cause more damage than x rays do, the dose equivalent incorporates the QF to account for the differences in biological effectiveness among the different radiations for monitoring purposes.

The concepts of dose equivalent versus absorbed dose might be illustrated by considering the following: Two separate exposures, each with a *dose equivalent* of 250 *rem* (2.5 Sv) would be expected to produce the same biological damage regardless of the types of radiation composing the exposures. Recall that the rem (Sv) is a calculated value incorporating the absorbed dose (a measured quantity) and the quality factor for each type of radiation involved. The QF is the "great equalizer" when considering dose equivalent. By comparison, a *dose* of 250 *rad* (2.5 Gy) of two different known types of radiation would be expected to produce biological damage characteristic of each of the radiation types involved.

In summary, when considering the overall effects of more than one kind of radiation, the rem or Sv is used as the unit of DE. Discussion of biological effects caused by only one type of radiation requires the use of rad or Gy terminology. When considering only x rays for diagnostic radiology, it is acceptable to assume the following relationships:

1.0 R = 1.0 rad = 1.0 rem, and

2.58 C/kg = 0.01 Gy = 0.01 Sv

Table 4–1 lists three types of ionizing radiations and the QF and DE for each type. Note that protons and alpha particles, which are types of particulate ionizing radiation, have much higher quality factors than x rays do. Protons are 10 times and alpha particles are 20 times more effective than x rays at producing a given biological effect at the same absorbed dose. Also note how the calculated value of the DE is affected by the value of the QF for the same absorbed dose of each type of radiation.

SOURCES OF RADIATION EXPOSURE

An individual is exposed to different types of radiation simply by existing from day to day. Radiation exposure encountered in daily life is referred to as *background radiation.* Some of the sources of background radiation are avoidable and others are not. The sources of background exposure can be divided into two major categories: *natural* and *artificial,* or manufactured. Since several kinds of radiation are responsible for background radiation exposure, and both somatic and genetic tissues must be assumed to have been exposed, the unit used to express the background dose must account for these factors. The dose equivalent (DE), as previously discussed, accounts for the relative effectiveness of different types of radiation to produce a certain biological response. The various somatic and genetic tissues possess their own degree of sensitivity to the different types of radiation encountered. Each of the various somatic and genetic tissues has been assigned a *tissue-weighting factor* that ranks each tissue relative to its risk or susceptibility to damage from a certain type of exposure. Additionally, background exposure is expressed as an annual quantity for a person living in the United States. Background exposure from all sources of radiation results in an *average*

Table 4–1. Dose Equivalent (DE) Calculations

Radiation	Absorbed Dose		Quality Factor		Dose Equivalent
In Rem (Standard System)					
X rays	5 rad	×	1	=	5 rem
Protons	5 rad	×	10	=	50 rem
Alpha particles	5 rad	×	20	=	100 rem
In Sv (International System)					
X rays	5 Gy	×	1	=	5 Sv
Protons	5 Gy	×	10	=	50 Sv
Alpha particles	5 Gy	×	20	=	100 Sv

annual effective dose of 3.60 mSv. The term "effective dose" results from the sum of the equivalent doses (DE) to each tissue multiplied by each tissue's weighting factor.

Natural background radiation exposure results from radon, cosmic radiation, terrestrial radiation, and internal source radiation. Artificial or manufactured background radiation exposure results from medical diagnostic and treatment modalities, consumer and industrial products, and other sources. Table 4–2 portrays the radiation sources, their respective annual effective dose, and the percentage of exposure from each source.

Radon occurs naturally as a solid, but since it is a radioactive material it undergoes a decay or breakdown process. One of the breakdown products of solid radon is radon gas. Radon becomes a contributor to natural background radiation exposure when its gas is taken into the lungs. While the gas is in the lungs it can decay to its next stage, which is a solid product, and remain in the lungs for an extended period of time. The result is chronic internal radiation exposure of the lung.

Levels of cosmic and terrestrial radiation are measured in air. Cosmic radiation originates in outer space from certain activities of the sun and other galactic and atmospheric phenomena. The quantity of cosmic radiation ultimately reaching the earth—and capable of being measured—is modified by altitude, latitude, barometric pressure, and solar activity. A person's effective dose from exposure to cosmic radiation can be influenced by the time spent in a building or outside, e.g., daily job conditions; by the number of airplane flights taken per year; or where a person lives. Structural shielding can modify an exposure from cosmic radiation by as much as 10%. A greater exposure will be experienced by someone living in Denver, Colorado, than by someone living at sea level.

Although structural shielding may reduce exposure to cosmic radiation, the shielding or building materials themselves may contribute to the levels of background exposure from terrestrial radiation. Terrestrial radiation depends on the type of soil and geographic location; thus, a brick or concrete building will emit a quantity of terrestrial radiation consistent with its geographic

Table 4–2. Average Annual Effective Dose of Ionizing Radiation from All Sources to a Member of the United States Population

Natural Sources	mSv	%
Radon	2.00	55.00
Cosmic	0.27	8.00
Terrestrial	0.28	8.00
Internal	0.39	11.00
Artificial, or Manufactured, Sources		
Medical applications		
Medical x rays	0.39	11.00
Dental x rays	0.01	0.30
Nuclear medicine	0.14	4.00
Consumer products	0.10	3.00
Other Sources		
Occupational	<0.01	<0.03
Nuclear fuel	<0.01	<0.03
Nuclear fallout	<0.01	<0.03
TOTAL	3.60 mSv	100%

location and the chemical composition of its construction materials. Soil naturally contains radium, thorium, and uranium and their decay products, as well as potassium-40.

Breathing the air and ingesting food are the most common routes of administration for many of the internal sources of radiation exposure. Exposure by an internal source of radiation requires the inhalation or ingestion of naturally occurring radionuclides and their isotopes. Included among these elements are thorium and uranium and their decay products, as well as tritium, carbon-14, and potassium-40, among others.

In addition to the naturally occurring radionuclides are cesium-137 and strontium-90, both of which have resulted from nuclear fallout. Of the two, strontium-90 causes the greatest concern because it is a pure beta-emitter (a particulate radiation) and has binding characteristics similar to those of calcium. Strontium-90 can become incorporated into developing teeth and bones as readily as calcium and may remain bound and active for 20 years or more.

Medical diagnosis and treatment modalities contribute the major percentage of manufactured radiation, whereas the combination of consumer and industrial sources and products contributes the smallest amount. The total exposure from medical applications of ionizing radiation is about 11%; dentistry accounts for about 3% of this total, or approximately 0.01 mSv.

OCCUPATIONAL AND NONOCCUPATIONAL RADIATION EXPOSURE

A person involved with the use of ionizing radiation as a part of professional responsibilities is classified as an *occupationally exposed person*. All other persons are considered *nonoccupationally exposed individuals* for radiation protection purposes. Annual dose limits have been established for both groups of the population, as well as for pregnant women. The dose limits set for nonoccupational and pregnant individuals are one tenth the dose for occupational radiation users. The National Council on Radiation Protection and Measurements (NCRP) has defined these dose limits within the context of the *Maximum Permissible Dose,* or MPD concept: "The MPD is the maximum dose of radiation that, in light of present knowledge, would not be expected to produce any significant radiation effects in a lifetime."

The MPD is quantified as the maximum dose equivalent (DE) that a person or a specified part thereof shall be allowed to receive in a stated period of time. The units of the MPD are the sievert and rem. Reassessment of the dosimetry data from the atomic bomb survivors and other highly exposed populations, along with an increased understanding of the nature and behavior of ionizing radiation, has resulted in several reductions in the MPD since the 1930s. In the 1990s, an occupationally exposed individual is allowed to receive a whole-body exposure of 20 mSv per year, based on a linear, non-threshold dose-response model (Fig. 4–1). Such a model states that even the smallest dose of radiation may have a damaging effect. The implications of this relationship are that no dose of radiation should be considered safe, that imaging techniques should be designed to provide a diagnostic image using the lowest possible dose, and that all unnecessary radiation exposure should be avoided. These points are embodied in the current philosophy of radiation use and protection and are summarized in the *ALARA* (*As Low As Reasonably Achievable*) *principle,* which calls for using the smallest amount of radiation practical to generate images of diagnostic quality.

EXPOSURE AND DOSE FROM ORAL AND MAXILLOFACIAL DIAGNOSTIC IMAGING

Negative effects of low-dose exposure to ionizing radiation are not readily demonstrable. Potential effects must be extrapolated as a statistical increase in the frequency of normally occurring disease states in the general population. The specific areas of concern for protection from excess exposure are the critical organs: bone marrow, thyroid gland, and gonads. The effective dose, as discussed earlier, is useful to compare doses from diagnostic radiation with the dose received from background radiation on a daily basis (Table 4–3).

Dose to the bone marrow is quantified as the *mean active bone marrow dose* in mSv. This dose is stated to be the average exposure distributed over all active bone marrow sites in the body. When considering exposure from intraoral and panoramic radiographs, the mandible is the primary active bone marrow site in the primary beam, although the mean active bone marrow dose from these techniques will be calculated to include all active marrow sites. The mean active bone marrow dose resulting from a full mouth intraoral survey of 20 films exposed using a rectangular or round collimator is 0.06 mSv and 0.142 mSv, respectively. The effective bone marrow dose for a survey taken with rectangular collimation is 0.033 mSv and is equivalent to 1 to 4 days of background radiation exposure. Round collimation results in

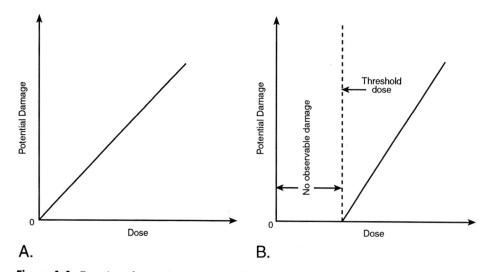

Figure 4–1. Genetic and somatic exposure. *A,* Exposure of genetic tissues is subject to a linear, nonthreshold dose-response model, which assumes that potential damage will occur at any dose; no dose is considered safe relative to genetic exposure. *B,* Somatic tissues generally respond according to a linear, threshold dose-response model, which illustrates that a certain minimal dose must be attained or exceeded before observable damage will occur.

an effective bone marrow dose of 0.084 mSv, or 4 to 10 days of background exposure.

The thyroid gland should always be protected from needless exposure to ionizing radiation by use of a thyroid collar. The x-ray dose to the thyroid gland from a 20-film full mouth survey is approximately 0.94 mGy and for a panoramic radiograph, about 0.74 mGy. Note that the units, mGy (mrad),

Table 4–3. Absorbed Dose, Effective Dose, and Equivalent Background Exposure from Common Dental Radiographic Procedures

Procedure	Film Type	Collimation	Absorbed Dose (mrad)	Effective Dose (mSv)	Background Equivalent
Full mouth (20 films)	E	Rectangular	16.1	0.033	1–2 days
	E	Round	51.4	0.084	4–5 days
	D	Rectangular			3–4 days
	D	Round			7–10 days
Bitewings (4 films)	E	Rectangular	3.1	0.007	7–10 hours
	E	Round	19.5	0.017	15–24 hours
	D	Rectangular			15–24 hours
	D	Round			24–48 hours
Panoramic	Rare earth screens		2.9	0.007	10–12 hours
	Calcium tungstate screens				24 hours

Note that using D-speed film or a calcium tungstate screen/film combination results in approximately twice the equivalent background exposure of E-speed film or rare earth screen/film systems.

express the radiation dose absorbed directly by the specific organ of concern, as compared with the mean bone marrow dose, expressed in mSv (mrem), which involves the units of the dose equivalent.

The reproductive organs are far removed from the site of dental radiographic procedures, but unnecessary exposure of the gonads results from scatter radiation from the patient's face if a lead apron is not used. One unavoidable but extremely minimal source of exposure to the gonads from dental radiography is the downward scatter of radiation through the patient's body. Because of the internal location of the female reproductive tissues, a slightly higher dose is received when compared with the gonads of males. Maximal reduction of the possibility of administering a genetically significant dose will be achieved by using a lead apron and thyroid collar on all patients for all oral and maxillofacial radiographic procedures.

Table 4–3 indicates that the absorbed dose from a full mouth survey of 20 E-speed films exposed using round collimation is approximately three times greater than when a rectangular collimator is in place on the x-ray machine tubehead. The effective doses and equivalent background exposure rates to critical organs are also proportionately greater with round collimation.

A panoramic radiograph taken with a rare earth screen exposes a patient to five times less radiation than a full mouth survey taken using rectangular collimation, and 17 times less than when a round collimator is employed. An interproximal survey consisting of four E-speed bitewings made with a round collimator and a panoramic radiograph made using a rare earth screen imparts one half the absorbed dose compared with a full mouth survey exposed with a round collimator.

Because of the length of time a panoramic machine takes to complete its excursion, patients often express concern about how great a dose they may have received. A meaningful comparison is that the dose from a panoramic radiograph made with rare earth screens is approximately equal to four E-speed bitewing radiographs. Absorbed doses are approximately twice as great when using D-speed film for intraoral radiography or exposing a panoramic radiograph with calcium tungstate screens.

Although intraoral direct digital imaging can result in significant dose reductions compared with film-based radiography, it must be kept in mind that intraoral digital image receptors are often smaller than the typical intraoral film that would have been selected for the same imaging task. A particular intraoral view made with a typical CCD may result in the need for additional exposures to cover the anatomical area of interest adequately. The total dose from multiple digital exposures may equal or even exceed that of a film-based examination.

RISK FROM DENTAL DIAGNOSTIC RADIOGRAPHY

Estimation of *risk* from exposure to ionizing radiation can be expressed as *absolute* or *relative* risk. The difference in risk between an irradiated population and a nonirradiated population defines absolute risk. Absolute risk is the additional risk resulting from an exposure to radiation and is expressed as:

the number of excess cancers beyond those that would occur spontaneously, per million persons, per rad, per year.

Absolute risk estimates for dental radiography are based on per million intraoral examinations made per year. Each million interproximal examinations using D-speed film and four bitewings might be expected to induce approximately 30 extra cancers over the life span of the persons irradiated. For every million full mouth surveys exposed using D-speed film, 100 extra cancers may be expected to occur among that population. If E-speed film or direct digital imaging is used, the risk is significantly reduced. Risk from dental radiographic procedures is stated as absolute risk.

The use of cancer as an indicator of excess risk assumes that cancer induction is equated to death from cancer. Distribution of excess cancers per million full mouth examinations has been estimated to occur as follows:

Thyroid cancer	**40%**
Malignant salivary gland cancer	**39%**
Leukemias	**13%**
Brain tumors	**6%**
Esophageal cancers	**2%**

Relative risk is the ratio of the risk for an irradiated or nonirradiated population. Relative risk is based on the statistical likelihood that a relationship will or will not exist between irradiation and cancer and is expressed as the term "r." When r is ≤ 1.0, there is no statistical association between irradiation and cancer. Relative risk of $r > 1.0$ indicates that a relationship exists between the irradiation and cancer. The association between irradiation and cancer becomes stronger the higher the r value becomes. Relative risk for ionizing radiation has a range of 1.0 to 9.5. An example of a relative risk is an r value of 1.75, which indicates that the exposed person will have a 75% higher risk of developing cancer than an unexposed individual.

EFFECTS OF IONIZING RADIATION ON LIVING SYSTEMS

Before entering into a discussion of the biological effects of ionizing radiation on living systems, it is necessary to recall the comments made at the beginning of this chapter about the sources of data from which radiobiological knowledge has been gained. Information on the human effects of radiation exposure has come from the analysis of unfortunate populations who were inadvertently exposed to high doses of ionizing radiation.

Diagnostic imaging, especially in dentistry, depends on low doses and infrequent exposures to accomplish its tasks. It is not possible to demonstrate directly that ionizing radiation in the *diagnostic energy range* causes untoward effects in human populations. The reason for this is that humans cannot be subjected to studies involving exposure to ionizing radiation. Computer simulation of x-ray interactions within human forms and extrapolation of the high-dose data from earlier human populations suggest that damage from low-dose exposures is a possibility. The uncertainty resulting from the lack of direct research data on human exposure to low-dose diagnostic radiation, and the suggestions of extrapolated data from populations exposed to high doses, have resulted in the radiation safety principles used today to minimize patient and operator exposure.

Effects on Biological Molecules

INDIRECT EFFECTS

Approximately 80% of the human body is water. It is no wonder, then, that the water molecule is the compound most often involved in radiation-induced biological effects. When energy from an x-ray beam interacts with a water molecule or some other abundantly occurring biomolecule, an *indirect action* of radiation is said to have occurred. Water is a relatively simple biomolecule that, when disrupted by radiation, can interact with other water molecules and with other either simple or more complex biomolecules. A water molecule that has been dissociated by an interaction with x radiation is said to have undergone the process of *radiolysis*. The reactive products of a dissociated water molecule are called *free radicals*. When a free radical combines with another biomolecule, the functional capacity of that biomolecule will be altered. Affected biomolecules are no longer capable of performing their normal function and can be considered "functionally dead." Since free radicals and altered biomolecules can migrate freely through the tissues of the organism, indirect effects of radiation can be manifested at sites distant from the original exposure.

The indirect effects of radiation occur far more often than *direct effects;* in fact, about two thirds of the biological damage caused by x rays is due to their indirect action.

DIRECT EFFECTS

For a direct effect of radiation to occur, an incident x-ray photon must interact directly with a biomolecule such as a protein, carbohydrate, lipid, and so on. The most significant biomolecule that could be affected by x radiation is DNA, a nucleic acid. A directly ionizing event may break the DNA strand or rearrange the base sequence.

Direct effects, indirect effects, the quality factor (QF), and relative biological effectiveness (RBE) are related by the concept of *linear energy transfer* (LET). LET is a measure of the rate at which energy is transferred from the incident radiation to the tissue along the path the radiation is traveling. The more energy transferred to the tissue per micrometer (μm) of travel, the higher the LET and the greater the tissue damage. For purposes of linear energy transfer, radiation is again classified as electromagnetic or particulate. X rays have a relatively low LET when compared with particulate radiation. Since x rays exhibit low LET, they are classified as *sparsely ionizing* radiation because they ionize relatively few atoms and/or biomolecules as they pass through a tissue. Protons and alpha particles are particulate radiation that exhibits high LET and generates many ionizing events as it traverses a tissue; this is called *densely ionizing* radiation. LET accounts for the ability of a certain type of radiation to produce a particular biological response. High LET radiation is more likely to cause a direct biological effect than low LET radiation.

Radiation protection applications use LET values when determining the quality factor (QF) used to calculate the dose equivalent (DE) for a particular type of radiation.

Effects on Cells

The sensitivity of cells to damage or death from radiation exposure depends on several factors. The LET of the radiation is a major determinant of lethality to the cell. A single, high LET photon that interacts with a vital biomolecule in the cell may cause sufficient damage to kill the cell. Cells may undergo *sublethal damage* if exposed to a low LET radiation, or if a high LET radiation interacts with a biomolecule that is abundant in the cell or is of minimal importance to the survival of the cell. Cells can recover from sublethal damage up to a point. The temperature and oxygen concentration of the environment surrounding the cells influence the degree of damage an exposure to radiation may cause. An environment of higher temperature or higher oxygen concentration will increase a cell's sensitivity to radiation. In either case, less of any type of radiation is required to produce a negative effect.

The age of the cells and whether they are part of a large or small volume of tissue influence their degree of radiosensitivity. The younger a cell, the more sensitive it is to the negative effects of radiation. The larger the volume of tissue that is irradiated, the more profound are the negative consequences for the entire organism. When a patient receives a dose of therapeutic radiation to a defined region of the head and neck to treat a carcinoma of the tongue, the effects of the exposure will be limited to the structures exposed by the beam of radiation. If the same dose applied to this limited area were spread out to cover the entire body, the results would be fatal.

Certain chemicals can influence the cellular response to radiation. Chemicals called *sensitizing agents* may double a cell's sensitivity to a dose of radiation. Put another way, only half the original dose of radiation may be necessary to cause a particular effect after a sensitizing agent has been administered. Sensitizing agents include vitamin K and actinomycin D, among others. The presence of another group of chemicals called *radioprotectors* results in doubling the required radiation dose to produce a particular effect after administration of the agent. Amifostine and sulfhydryl compounds such as cysteine act as radioprotectors.

The amount of radiation administered over a period of time, or the *dose rate,* affects a cell's response to the exposure. Dose rates generally can be classified as *acute, protracted,* and *fractionated.* A dose of 1.0 Gy (100 rad) given all at once, defined as an acute radiation exposure, exhibits the most profound effects whether given as a local or a whole-body exposure, and this dose is the maximum rate at which a dose can be given. Lowering of the dose rate can be accomplished by dose protraction or fractionation. A protracted dose of 1.0 Gy will be administered at some constant amount, say 0.01 Gy, over a specified period of time until the total dose has been given. A fractionated dose of 1.0 Gy would be given in several equal doses separated by specific time intervals until the entire dose has been applied. Dose protraction and fractionation take advantage of a cell's ability to repair sublethal damage. Manipulation of tissue temperature and oxygen concentration, tissue volume irradiated, dose rate and the administration of chemical sensitizers are employed in radiation therapy to enhance killing of neoplastic cells while giving healthy cells the opportunity to recover.

Neoplastic cells generally are very young and actively dividing cells. The *law of Bergonié and Tribondeau* states that actively proliferating, poorly differentiated cells or those with a large nucleus to cytoplasm ratio, and cells that will undergo many more divisions in their lifetime, are the most sensitive to radiation. The law of Bergonié and Tribondeau has a few exceptions, most notably the mature lymphocyte. This cell is highly differentiated and will not divide, but it has a large nucleus to cytoplasm ratio and is highly sensitive to radiation.

There are times during the life cycle of a cell during which it is most vulnerable to the negative effects of radiation. Interphase is the period of a cell's life when it is growing and preparing to divide by mitosis. Interphase is composed of three components: the G_1 phase during which cell growth actually occurs; the S phase, described as the time when DNA is synthesized; and the G_2 phase in which the biomolecules needed for mitosis are assembled. Cells are most resistant to radiation during the S phase of the interphase and most sensitive during mitosis or while they are dividing. Cancer radiotherapy is effective because neoplastic cells are immature, undifferentiated cells that are undergoing many divisions or mitoses.

A cell may undergo chromosome damage by an exposure to radiation. Although chromosomes are subject to spontaneous breaks, radiation can increase the frequency or severity of the break. Most of the time the broken pieces will adhere to each other and will be reattached and repaired. If an exposure to radiation occurs during mitosis and while the chromosomes are in motion, the detached pieces may become separated and a repair may not occur. Multiple chromosome breaks can result in rearrangement of genetic components, altered gene sequencing, and an abnormally functioning cell. These cells usually die during their next mitosis. A list of cell types of the body and their radiosensitivities is provided in Table 4–4.

Effects on Tissues, Organs, and Systems

The human organism follows an orderly progression in complexity, beginning with subatomic particles and building on these to synthesize atoms,

Table 4–4. Ranges of Cell Radiosensitivity

Degree of Radiosensitivity	Cell Type
High	Lymphocytes Spermatogonia Erythroblasts Intestinal crypt cells
Intermediate	Endothelial cells Osteoblasts Spermatids Fibroblasts
Low	Muscle cells Nerve cells Chondrocytes

molecules, cells, tissues, organs, and systems. When radiation damages a sufficient quantity of any of these components, the continuum is disrupted and the effects of the exposure become evident. A localized therapeutic dose of radiation affects all components of the continuum lying in the path of the beam. A whole-body exposure of the same dose will affect all components of the body and will most likely be fatal. The most radiosensitive cells in the path of the beam determine the intensity of the negative response to the exposure. Localized therapeutic doses and whole-body exposure to high levels of radiation result in *early* and *late effects.*

EARLY EFFECTS

Whole-Body Exposure

Death is the ultimate early effect from an acute, whole-body exposure to a high dose of radiation. Depending on the level of the dose received, different groups of symptoms appear at somewhat specific time intervals. These dose-related symptoms are referred to as *acute radiation syndrome.* A high-level whole-body dose such as 1.0 Gy (100 rad) or more is usually sufficient to cause death in several days to weeks. The acute radiation syndrome involves the hematological, gastrointestinal, and nervous systems. Before the symptoms from high-dose exposure of these systems appear, there is a *prodromal period* beginning in minutes to hours after the exposure and lasting for hours to days. The acute prodromal symptoms consist of nausea, vomiting, and diarrhea, with their severity depending on the size of the dose. The prodromal period ends and the person feels fine, again for a length of time lasting from hours for extremely high dose exposures to weeks for lesser doses. This period of apparent wellness is referred to as the *latent period.*

Following the latent period, the symptoms of the acute radiation syndrome reappear, and the damage to specific organ systems becomes apparent. Organ systems with the most immature and most frequently dividing cell populations are affected first. As dose levels increase, the damage becomes evident in the relatively more resistant systems in addition to the already affected tissues and organs. Extremely high exposure levels cause death in so short a time that the prodromal and latent periods may be extremely short or nonexistent, and hematological and gastrointestinal symptoms may not have a chance to develop. In these cases the patient usually dies from central nervous system damage and respiratory arrest within a matter of a few hours after the exposure.

The *hematological syndrome,* which involves the highly radiosensitive cells of the bone marrow, usually results from a whole-body dose in the range of 2 to 10 Gy (200 to 1000 rad). The prodromal and latent periods may last up to 4 weeks. Since the blood-forming tissues of the bone marrow were damaged or destroyed by the radiation, all cellular elements of the blood are decreasing during this time. The decrease in all types of circulating blood cells causes a return of the nausea, vomiting, and diarrhea, accompanied now by lethargy, malaise, and fever. Blood components continue to decline in number if the dose was lethal, and the patient will die from infection, hemorrhage, dehydration, and electrolyte imbalance. Recovery in several weeks to months is possible if the dose was not lethal.

Symptoms of the *gastrointestinal syndrome* begin to appear after about 10 to 50 Gy (1000 to 5000 rad) of whole-body exposure. The prodromal period may begin within hours of the exposure and last for 24 to 36 hours. The relatively symptom-free latent period may last for 3 to 5 days—about the length of time it takes for the intestinal lining present before the exposure to be lost. The radiation kills the highly proliferative intestinal crypt cells that are responsible for the continuous replacement of the intestinal lining every 3 to 5 days. Nausea, vomiting, and diarrhea reappear, along with persistent hematological symptoms, owing to a progressive decrease in circulating blood cells. The severity of the diarrhea results in complete loss of the intestinal lining, and death follows in about a week from hemorrhage, dehydration, and electrolyte imbalance.

Death usually follows a whole-body exposure of more than 50 Gy (5000 rad) in a matter of a few hours or days. The person experiences almost immediate nausea, followed by excitation, confusion, loss of vision, a burning sensation or tingling of the skin, and eventual loss of consciousness. This group of symptoms constitutes the *central nervous system syndrome*. During a short latent period of 6 to 12 hours the damage progresses and the symptoms return. The person most likely becomes disoriented and experiences loss of muscle control and balance, accompanied by respiratory distress, seizures, coma, and death. After a dose of this magnitude, the hematological and gastrointestinal systems have been irreversibly damaged, but the person will have died before related symptoms can develop.

Localized or Restricted Exposure

Radiation therapy often employs exposure to doses of the same magnitude as discussed in the previous section. The restricted area of therapeutic exposures and other modifying factors such as dose rate allow high doses to be administered with beneficial effects. An accidental, acute high-dose exposure to a localized area will damage the tissues in the path of the beam but is not likely to be fatal.

The skin commonly exhibits the early radiation effect of *erythema* when overexposed to the sun's rays. A single x-ray dose of 3 to 10 Gy (300 to 1000 rad) may produce erythema in 24 to 36 hours in the area of skin exposed. There is then a latent period of about 2 weeks during which the redness and burning subside. The redness and burning then return with greater intensity, followed by desquamation or loss of skin in the irradiated area (Fig. 4–2). The skin also may undergo *epilation,* or hair loss, when exposed to a sufficient dose of radiation; changes in skin pigmentation may occur in association with loss of fingernails (Fig. 4–3).

When a person undergoes radiation therapy for cancer in the head and neck region, all the cell and tissue types in the path of the beam will be affected. These include the skin, salivary glands, muscles, bone, blood vessels, nerves, intraoral mucosa, taste buds, developing teeth, and so on. Radiation will have a direct negative effect on some of these structures, but others will be secondarily affected. Radiotherapeutic doses to the head and neck, although fractionated and otherwise controlled, are often in the range of 40 to 50 Gy (4000 to 5000 rad) and produce significant early effects in these local structures.

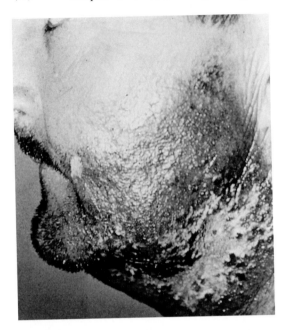

Figure 4-2. Desquamation of the skin over the side of the face and neck.

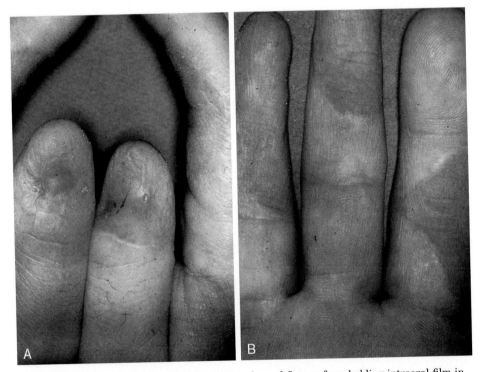

Figure 4-3. Chronic long-term exposure of thumbs and fingers from holding intraoral film in patients' mouths during exposures. *A,* Loss of thumbnails due to destruction of the proliferative cells in the nailbed. *B,* Accompanying increased pigmentation and alteration of skin texture on flexor surfaces of fingers.

The skin of the face and neck on the side of the radiation source will undergo erythema and its sequelae once the dose has exceeded about 3 to 6 Gy (300 to 600 rad). The intraoral mucosa can be affected by doses as low as 1 to 3 Gy (100 to 300 rad). Early signs include erythema and edema and may occur after only 1 or 2 days of therapy. This is the condition known as *radiation mucositis,* and it may persist for several weeks (Fig. 4–4). Radiation mucositis can become very painful, and after about 2 weeks of radiation treatment patients may have a difficult time speaking, eating, and swallowing. If teeth are present, brushing and flossing can be very painful, but in the radiation therapy patient excellent oral hygiene is a requirement. It is sometimes recommended that all teeth be extracted prior to radiotherapy to avoid the difficulties inherent in maintaining the teeth after treatment. Edentulous persons often have comparable difficulty wearing appliances due to the tender tissue under the appliance.

A major factor contributing to the painful mucosa, the difficulties in oral hygiene, and the wearing of tissue-borne appliances is *xerostomia,* a condition in which the quantity of saliva is diminished. In xerostomia associated with radiation therapy, not only is the amount of saliva decreased but also it is more viscous and has a more acid pH. The diminished quantity and increased viscosity of the saliva detract from the lubricating function it once performed. Normal saliva also functions to keep debris from adhering to the teeth, a function much diminished after radiotherapy. The dry and fragile mucosa, scant quantity, and highly viscous, slightly acidic saliva make the intraoral environment ideal for the overgrowth of certain normal flora and supportive of the growth of acidogenic organisms not normally present. The mucosa becomes particularly susceptible to infection by normally nonthreatening

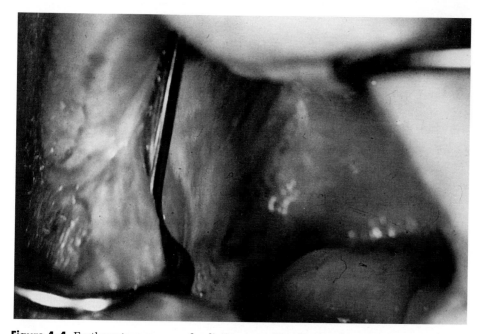

Figure 4–4. Erythematous mucosa of radiation mucositis affecting the right posterior buccal mucosa and retromolar pad areas beyond the cheek retractor.

microorganisms. Acidogenic organisms thrive in the new environment, plaque tends to accumulate more rapidly and adhere to the teeth more tenaciously, and caries rapidly can become rampant.

Caries in the patient undergoing radiotherapy are often erroneously called *radiation caries*. Caries associated with radiation therapy occur secondarily to exposure of the salivary glands and the subsequent alterations of the saliva previously discussed. Three types of radiation caries can be seen clinically. The most common presentation is rampant caries affecting all surfaces of the teeth. The unusual features of this presentation are that cusp tips, incisal edges, and smooth enamel surfaces devoid of pits or other discontinuities can become carious. Another type of caries associated with radiotherapy is sometimes called *amputation caries* (Fig. 4–5). These lesions involve the cementum and dentin in the cervical region and may progress around the circumference of the tooth, resulting in loss or "amputation" of the crown. Third, the crowns of exposed teeth may take on a dark appearance and be subject to accelerated incisal or occlusal wear.

Radiation damage to developing teeth is dose dependent. Exposure to therapeutic doses before calcification may destroy the tooth bud. Irradiation following the start of calcification may affect cellular differentiation and result in malformed teeth. Children irradiated for a head and neck neoplasm may present with permanent teeth exhibiting retarded root development, dwarfed

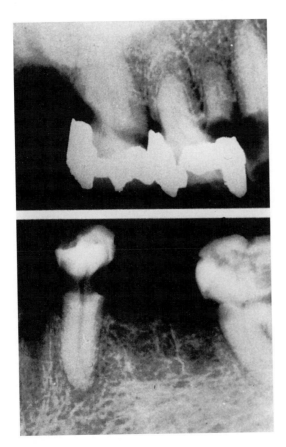

Figure 4–5. So-called "amputation" caries, a possible sequela of radiation therapy during which the salivary glands were irradiated. The crowns of the teeth can be "amputated" from their roots by this caries process.

teeth, or failure of one or more tooth buds to form teeth. Irradiation of partly developed teeth may or may not stop the process and may cause premature eruption. Although exposure of developing teeth may hinder or halt their root development, the eruptive mechanism is essentially unaffected and teeth having bizarre root forms will still erupt (Fig. 4–6).

Taste buds are radiosensitive. During the second or third week of radiotherapy, patients will experience a loss of taste discrimination. The degree of collimation of the therapeutic beam may be useful in predicting the extent of the effects of the dose regimen. When the posterior two thirds of the tongue is irradiated, bitter and acid flavors will be less appreciated. Sweet and salty flavors will be diminished when the anterior one third of the tongue receives the exposure. Accompanying alterations of the saliva may contribute to the loss of taste acuity. The ability to taste usually returns to nearly normal after 60 to 120 days.

Muscles are among the more radioresistant tissues, but direct exposure to the primary beam will result in damage to the muscle cells. Of equal or greater significance to exposure of the muscle cells is the exposure of the blood vessels feeding the muscles. These small vessels are referred to as *fine vasculature* and are intermediate in their sensitivity to radiation exposure. Radiation damage of the fine vasculature causes them to degenerate and results in a loss of blood flow to the muscle tissues. Without nutrients, the muscles begin to atrophy and shrink. The nutrition of the patient may be severely compromised, and physical therapy should be part of the recovery plan.

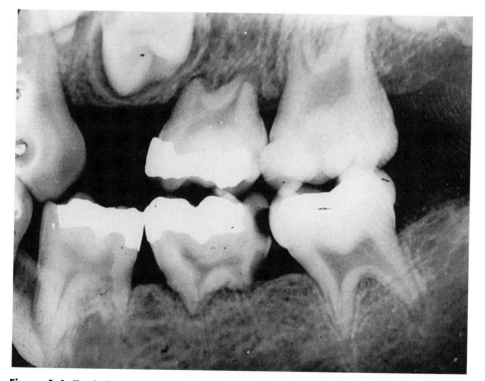

Figure 4–6. Teeth that have bizarre root forms may erupt if subjected to radiation during their development.

Bone, like muscle, is usually in the path of the primary beam in head and neck radiotherapy. The mandible is the bone of chief concern. The vascular supply to the mandible is somewhat sparse to begin with but especially when considering the fine vasculature. Irradiation of the mandible will result in its bone marrow becoming hypovascular, hypoxic, and hypocellular. Normal bone marrow contains a rich supply of immature and highly proliferative blood-forming cells. Irradiation can cause these cells to diminish in number and the normal marrow to be replaced by fat or fibrous connective tissue. The normal activity of bone turnover mediated by osteoblasts and osteoclasts may be brought to a halt, and necrosis may begin.

Bone subjected to doses in the range of 50 to 60 Gy or more is especially susceptible to infection by bacterial organisms normally present in the mouth. An incident of minor mucosal trauma or active periapical or periodontal disease may allow normal microorganisms to penetrate the soft tissues and enter the bone. The resulting infection of the bone is termed *osteoradionecrosis*. Such infections can be acute or chronic, are extremely difficult to eradicate, and remain a lifelong threat for these patients. The compromised status of postirradiated bone is a paramount reason for the need of a dental evaluation, a concise treatment plan, and definitive treatment directed at the elimination of local irritating factors and dental disease prior to the initiation of radiotherapy to the head and neck.

LATE EFFECTS

Late effects of radiation are those that become apparent several months or years following the exposure. The two categories of late effects are *genetic* and *somatic* (see Fig. 4–1). Genetic effects include alteration of chromosomes that may result in mutations in future generations. Genetic effects are believed to occur according to a *linear, nonthreshold* dose-response model. Such a model implies that no dose of radiation is safe when considering genetic information to be passed on to future generations. Somatic effects include cancer and other disorders that do not involve the reproductive or genetic tissues. Somatic effects generally follow a *linear, threshold* dose-response model. This relationship states that a certain minimal dose (threshold dose) is necessary before demonstrable damage will occur, although a degree of cumulative damage ensues until the threshold dose is reached or exceeded. Various somatic tissues are designated as *critical organs,* thus giving rise to the *Critical Organ Concept* (Table 4–5). *Carcinogenesis* is a late somatic effect of exposure to ionizing radiation and can affect most any tissue or organ in the body. Cancer caused by ionizing radiation appears no different from cancer that occurs spontaneously.

Data for estimating the risk or possible occurrence of late effects from exposure to high levels of ionizing radiation, other than radiotherapy, have come from studying various human populations. Those who survived the World War II atomic bomb blasts of Hiroshima and Nagasaki were assessed for the incidence of, or death from, breast or other types of cancer. Patients afflicted with ankylosing spondylitis and treated with radiation were evaluated for the occurrence of, or death from, leukemia or other cancers. Women who received fluoroscopic breast examinations were followed for the incidence

Table 4–5. Critical Organ Concept; Critical Organs and Potential Effects of Radiation

Organ	Effect
Female breast	Cancer
Skin	Cancer
Thyroid	Cancer
Lens of the eye	Cataracts
Bone marrow	Leukemia
Hematopoietic tissues and organs	Leukemia
Gonads	Mutations
	Impaired fertility
Fetus (pregnancy)	Developmental

of, or death from, breast cancer. Children irradiated to treat tinea capitis were assessed for the incidence of thyroid cancer.

The great majority of cancer occurs spontaneously. The death rate from cancer in the United States is approximately 20%, with a very small portion of the carcinogenesis being attributed to exposure to low-dose radiation. If an exposure above the diagnostic energy range occurs, most cancers will appear within 10 years of the exposure. An exposed person not developing cancer by the tenth year is presumed to carry the increased risk for a lifetime. An individual excessively exposed during childhood is subject to approximately twice the risk of an adult receiving the same dose. Cancers induced by radiation are considered to occur in addition to spontaneously occurring cancers. The number of radiation-induced cases is a multiple of the spontaneous cancer rate.

Following excessive exposure of the bone marrow, the incidence of leukemia and bone cancer usually increases within 5 years and tends to return to the spontaneous incidence rate within 30 years. The incidence rate of leukemia follows a linear-quadratic dose-response relationship. Such a relationship implies that at lower doses the incidence of leukemia increases in proportion (linearly) to each increase in dose, and as the dose continues to increase, the rate of leukemogenesis accelerates. Exposed persons under 20 years of age are susceptible to an increased risk for leukemia.

The thyroid gland is susceptible to an increased incidence of carcinoma following exposure to ionizing radiation. The likelihood of radiation-induced thyroid carcinogenesis is greater in childhood than at any other time during a person's life. Radiogenic as well as spontaneous thyroid cancer is two to three times more likely to occur in females than in males. Exposure of the thyroid gland can be reduced by 50 to 98% when the thyroid collar is used for dental radiographic procedures.

Tumors of the salivary glands have been shown to be more prevalent in the atomic bomb survivors, in persons who have received radiation treatment in which the salivary glands were in the path of the therapeutic beam, and in persons exposed to diagnostic levels of radiation. Diagnostic levels of x radiation in excess of 500 mGy to the head and neck region have been correlated with an increased incidence of parotid gland tumors. This increased risk is most likely to exist for individuals receiving several full mouth radiographic examinations before 20 years of age.

The brain and central nervous system are most susceptible to damage by ionizing radiation at a young age. In utero exposure to diagnostic x-ray studies increases the risk of mortality from brain tumors. Research has demonstrated an association between intracranial meningiomas and previous medical or several dental full mouth radiographic examinations before the age of 20 years. Mental retardation has a 4% chance of occurrence per 100 mSv of exposure during the gestational period of 8 to 15 weeks, and there is less risk from exposure during other gestational times. Fetal exposure from an average dental radiographic examination approaches 0.01 mSv when a lead apron and thyroid collar are used. According to the National Council of Radiation Protection and Measurements (NCRP) the likelihood of inducing congenital defects is negligible from gonadal doses below 5000 mrem (50 mSv). The relative risk of experiencing a first-generation birth defect from dental radiography has been shown to be 9 in 1 billion, or $9.0 \times 10^{-7}\%$.

The risk of impaired fertility or sterility from dental radiographic exposures is nil when the lead apron and thyroid collar are used. Although doses to the reproductive organs are extremely low even without the protection of a lead apron and thyroid collar, radiation safety principles state that the dose should be reduced as far as possible and still allow production of a diagnostic image. The effects on fertility are dose dependent and require a minimal threshold dose to be exceeded before damage is manifest.

Although cataracts of the lens of the eye require a significant threshold dose for occurrence, much higher than any routine dental diagnostic procedure would involve, the proximity of the eye to the structures treated by the dental team makes its mention worthwhile. The threshold dose necessary to initiate cataract formation is about 2 Gy (200 rad) when the radiation is given in a single exposure. The threshold rises to at least 5 Gy (500 rad) if the dose is received in multiple exposures over a period of weeks.

METHODS TO REDUCE EXPOSURE AND DOSE FROM DENTAL DIAGNOSTIC RADIOGRAPHY

The following methods to reduce patient radiation exposure and dose from dental radiography are discussed next.

        Patient selection criteria
        Image receptor type
        X-ray machine type
        Filtration
        Source-to-image receptor distance
        Collimation
        Lead apron and thyroid collar
        Quality assurance

Methods providing operator protection are also reviewed.

Patient Selection Criteria

Guidelines have been established for prescribing dental radiographs to help ensure the optimum use of ionizing radiation for diagnostic purposes. These guidelines are officially entitled *Guidelines for Prescribing Dental Radiographs** and are also known as *Patient Selection Criteria.* The intent of the guidelines is to eliminate so-called "routine" radiographic procedures based on nothing more than the same time intervals as recall visits. The guidelines are derived from descriptions of clinical situations composed of patient signs, symptoms, and history that require a radiographic examination to secure diagnostic information obtainable in no other way. The primary message of the guidelines is that before a radiographic examination is performed, the dentist should discuss the dental history with the patient to determine whether any unusual signs or symptoms are present and then should perform a clinical examination to detect any occult indications of the need for a radiographic examination. Radiographs to be taken should be prescribed based on the historical and clinical findings, i.e., whether a demonstrable clinical indication exists.

Consistent use of selection guidelines will help ensure that patient exposure and expense will be kept to a minimum and diagnostic yield will be maximal. Use of the recommendations may result in patients at low risk for dental disease receiving fewer radiographs and higher-risk individuals receiving more radiographs over time. The guidelines place patients into three broad categories based on the type of visit (new or recall), dental status (child, adolescent, adult), and risk (for caries and periodontal disease, and growth and development). The guidelines apply to pregnant women as well.

Children are considered to be in the primary dentition stage of development until eruption of the first permanent molars. The transitional phase of dental development begins with eruption of the first permanent tooth. Adolescents are defined as having all permanent teeth erupted except for the third molars. Adults are either dentulous or edentulous according to the guidelines.

New patients without previous radiographs should have surveys individually designed to assess historical and clinical findings. Recall patients may or may not present with historical or clinical indications requiring radiographic assessment. Periodontal disease or a history of periodontal disease in a new patient is a strong indication of the need for a radiographic evaluation. Assessment of growth and development and correlation of systemic disease with possible radiographic manifestations are additional considerations for prescribing a radiographic examination.

Following is a partial list of clinical situations for which radiographs may be indicated:

- **Positive historical findings**
  previous periodontal or endodontic treatment
  history of pain or trauma
  familial history of dental anomalies
  postoperative evaluation of healing
  presence of implants

---

*The monograph, *Guidelines for Prescribing Dental Radiographs,* is available from Eastman Kodak Company, Health Sciences Division, Rochester, NY. Publication Number N-80 A A8H017.

- **Positive clinical signs and/or symptoms**
  clinical evidence of periodontal disease
  large or deep restorations
  deep carious lesions
  malposed or clinically impacted teeth
  swelling
  evidence of facial trauma
  mobile teeth
  fistulous tracts or parulides
  growth abnormalities
  oral involvement by systemic disease
  temporomandibular joint pain or dysfunction
  facial asymmetry
  abutment teeth or potential abutment teeth

The following list enumerates some of the conditions with which a person at high risk for caries may present:

- high level of past caries activity

- poor condition of restorations

- history of inadequate fluoride

- high sucrose diet

- developmental defects of enamel

- history of radiation therapy

- history of recurrent caries

- poor oral hygiene

- history of prolonged nursing

- poor family dental health

- xerostomia

Professional judgment, patient concerns, economic factors, and medicolegal pressures are just a few of the elements that will influence the consistent application of patient selection criteria.

Image Receptor Type

Radiation safety principles favor the use of the fastest image receptor available. The fastest image recording medium consists of the variety of electronic image receptors discussed earlier. Radiation dose to critical organs in the head and neck region can be reduced by 80% or more when using electronic systems for intraoral techniques, compared with the fastest intraoral film available. Early studies utilizing digital examinations with storage phosphors for panoramic and cephalometric radiography have demonstrated a 40 to 60% mean dose reduction when compared with a standard screen-film combination.

The fastest intraoral film available is Ektaspeed Plus (Eastman Kodak Company, Rochester, New York), introduced in 1994. The physical characteristics of this film were discussed in Chapter 3. Ektaspeed Plus was immediately preceded by Ektaspeed, both of which are speed E film types. Ektaspeed film was preceded by Ultraspeed, a speed D film, and the two film types have been on the market concurrently for several years. Historically, Ultraspeed images have been perceived as sharper than Ektaspeed images. Several studies have demonstrated that images from both film types are comparable, although an optimal image with Ektaspeed depends more on strict processing quality control. The physical makeup of Ektaspeed and Ultraspeed was also discussed earlier.

Ektaspeed Plus has been shown to have contrast similar to that of Ultraspeed film, and of the three films is the least affected by variations in processing conditions. Early comparisons of the three film types suggest that clinicians who have continued to use Ultraspeed film, in spite of the need for twice the exposure time of a speed E film type, can now switch to a film that results in half the patient dose and produces high-quality diagnostic images throughout the effective life of the processing chemicals. Ektaspeed Plus is the fastest intraoral film available.

X-Ray Machine Type

Constant potential x-ray machines produce an x-ray beam consisting principally of high-frequency, short wavelength energy; thus shorter exposure times can be utilized. High kVp beams reduce patient dose and produce long scale, low-contrast images with many shades of gray that will provide maximum information about subtle changes in tissue densities.

Filtration

X-ray machines are installed with a mandated amount of total filtration, as discussed earlier. Several studies have addressed the use of rare earth intensifying screen material or after-market filter kits placed over the exit port of the x-ray machine tubehead to further reduce the number of low-energy photons reaching the patient. The addition of rare earth filtration material in the path of the beam has been shown to reduce patient exposure by 25 to 70%. Niobium filter material, for example, can decrease the skin surface exposure in the range of 40 to 50%.

Source-to-Image Receptor Distance

The distance of the x-ray source from the image receptor will influence patient dose. This distance, commonly referred to as the source-to-film distance (SFD), will affect the intensity of the x-ray beam that interacts with the patient and image receptor to create an image. Since beam intensity is directly related to radiographic density, changing the SFD will result in a concurrent change in beam intensity and in the density of the resultant radiograph according to the inverse square law.

The source-receptor distance should be as great as the radiographic system will permit. The distances used in association with intraoral radiography are determined in part by the length of the collimator attached to the machine tubehead. Eight and sixteen inches are the two most commonly used source-to-receptor distances. This distance for a particular machine is measured from the end of the collimator to a dot or similar marking on the tubehead casing, which indicates the location of the x-ray tube target inside the machine.

Additionally, a longer SFD results in a less divergent beam's exiting the collimator, and consequently a smaller area of the patient's face will be exposed. A sharper image with minimal magnification will also result from a longer SFD.

Operators must understand the relationship between the inverse square law and beam intensity, radiographic density, and exposure time to compensate for changes in SFD. The inverse square law states that the beam intensity is inversely related to the square of the source-to-film distance. It implies that radiographic (image) density is also inversely related to the square of source-to-film distance, since density is directly related to intensity. The purpose of applying the inverse square law when changing the SFD is to maintain the original radiographic density. The original density is maintained by adjusting the exposure time to compensate for the changes that will occur in intensity when the SFD is changed. The following simple rules can be applied to maintain density while changing the source-receptor distance. (Chapter 2 contains additional examples for application of the inverse square law.)

When the source-to-receptor distance is doubled, the original exposure time should be multiplied by four to maintain the original beam intensity and image density.

When the source-to-receptor distance is reduced by one half, one fourth of the original exposure time should be used to maintain the original beam intensity and image density.

Collimation

The use of a speed E film, patient selection criteria, lead apron and thyroid collar, and rectangular collimation (PID) with the greatest practical source-to-image receptor distance constitute the latest recommendations to minimize patient dose from intraoral dental radiography. The area of a patient's face exposed by the x-ray beam exiting from a round, lead-lined cylindrical collimator measuring 2.75 inch (7.0 cm) in diameter should be considered the maximum allowable area to be subjected to such an exposure. This area can be significantly reduced by replacing the round collimator with a rectangular aluminum PID (Fig. 4–7; see also Fig. 2–7). Several manufacturers make devices intended to reduce a round beam to a rectangular beam by clipping the device either to the end of the round collimator or to the ring of the paralleling instrument (Fig. 4–8). An aluminum rectangular collimator allows an area of skin only slightly larger than a number 2 periapical film to be

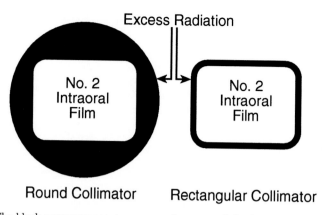

Figure 4–7. The black areas represent excess surface area of the face exposed each time a radiograph is made with a number 2 size intraoral film using round collimation and rectangular collimation. Rectangular collimation exposes approximately 60 to 70% less of a patient's face per film, which results in a significant reduction in total exposure for a full-mouth survey.

exposed. This translates into a 60 to 70% decrease in surface dose to a patient's face and a 45 to 95% overall dose reduction, depending on the anatomical site being radiographed.

Lead Apron and Thyroid Collar

The principal purpose of the lead apron is to protect the female breast and the reproductive and hematopoietic tissues from exposure to radiation scattered from the patient's face (Fig. 4–9). The proximity of the thyroid gland to the primary beam makes it susceptible not only to scatter from within the body, as mentioned earlier, but also to direct exposure from the divergent primary x-ray beam.

The mean gonadal dose per day from background radiation exposure is approximately 0.3 to 0.5 mrem (0.03 to 0.05 mSv). A full mouth survey of 20 films taken with a round collimator and without a lead apron covering the patient will result in a genetic dose of around 0.5 mrad (0.05 mGy). Rectangular collimation, even without a lead apron in place, would reduce this dose to 0.2 mrad (0.02 mGy). Using a lead apron with either type of collimation will reduce the genetic dose to a range of 0.01 to 0.03 mrad (0.001 to 0.003 mGy). The reader should recall the significant reduction in surface exposure to a patient's face when rectangular collimation is used.

The dose to the thyroid gland can be reduced by 50% or more when a thyroid collar is used. A standard full mouth survey (20 films) taken without a thyroid collar delivers a thyroid dose of 20 to 50 mrad (0.20 to 0.50 mGy), depending on the type of collimation used. Patients radiographed with a thyroid collar receive a thyroid dose ranging from 10 to 25 mrad (0.10 to 0.25 mGy). The threshold dose for the induction of thyroid cancer ranges from 5000 to 7000 mrem (50 to 70 mSv).

Radiographic examinations of pregnant women should be performed according to the recommendations set forth in the *Guidelines for Prescribing*

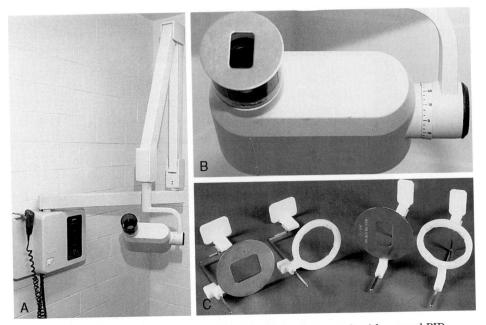

Figure 4–8. Clip-on rectangular collimators. *A,* An intraoral x-ray unit with a round PID (collimator) mounted on the machine tubehead. *B,* Rectangular collimator clipped to the end of a round, tubehead-mounted collimator. *C,* Anterior and posterior intraoral paralleling technique instruments with and without rectangular collimators attached.

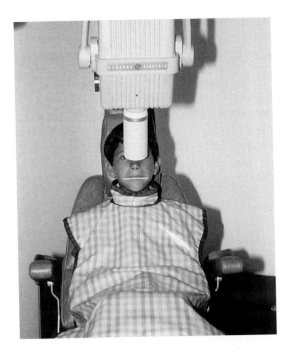

Figure 4–9. Proper use of a lead apron and thyroid collar for intraoral radiography.

Dental Radiographs. Placement of a lead apron and thyroid collar is mandatory, as for all patients. An additional protective measure advocated by some practitioners is to place a second lead apron over the patient's back, extending below the level of the fetus. The intent of this maneuver, although not substantiated by research findings, is to prevent possible fetal exposure from radiation scattered by the metal components of the chair. Recall that research has demonstrated gonadal exposure from dental radiographic procedures to be nil when a lead apron and thyroid collar are placed over the front of the patient, as is customary practice.

Panoramic radiography requires a specially designed lead apron that shields the patient's back and front as the machine completes its excursion. Panoramic systems do not allow a thyroid collar to be used because it will block a portion of the x-ray beam.

Lead aprons and thyroid collars should be handled with care. Rough handling, folding, or otherwise introducing creases into the lead apron or collar should be avoided. Repeated folding, bending, or creasing will result eventually in loss of continuity of the lead dispersed inside the apron or collar and a subsequent decrease in its ability to attenuate x rays. Lead aprons should not be folded and draped over towel bars but gently placed on hangers designed to support the weight of the apron. These hangers allow the apron to hang flat, with their weight borne by the shoulder area of the apron. Some aprons are supplied with loops to provide a means for proper weight distribution and hanging (Fig. 4–10).

Operator Protection

Operators of x-ray machines in dental practice must adhere to a few simple rules to keep their occupational exposure to a minimum. These radiation safety rules pertain to an operator's position relative to the sources of radiation in the operatory. Three sources of radiation exist in each operatory that houses an x-ray machine: (1) the primary beam of radiation as it exits from the collimator, (2) radiation potentially leaking from the tubehead during an exposure, and (3) scatter or secondary radiation from the patient's face.

Operators should never locate themselves in the path of the primary beam. In addition, operators should not position themselves on the same side of the patient on which the x-ray source is located. The primary beam is potentially the source of the greatest exposure to office staff involved in radiography. Scatter radiation from the surface of the patient nearest the x-ray source represents the second greatest potential source of operator exposure. Radiography staff should make every effort to position themselves behind a radiation-safe barrier during exposures. When a barrier is not available, the operator should be positioned at least 6 feet from the radiation source and the patient, and at an angle of from 90 to 135° to the path of the primary beam. Figure 4–11 illustrates the preferred operator positions in relation to the path of the primary beam and scatter radiation from the side of the patient nearest the source of radiation.

All office staff must be forbidden to hold films in a patient's mouth. In the event of an uncooperative child patient, the parent or guardian should be brought into the operatory, covered with a lead apron and thyroid collar, and

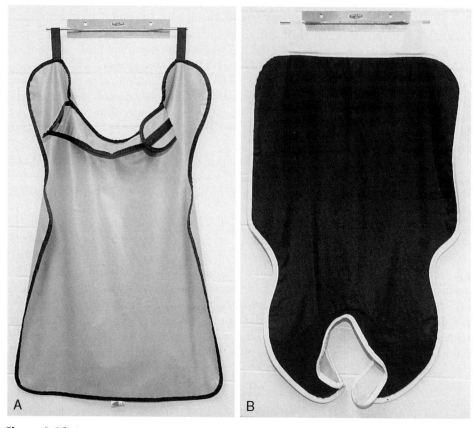

Figure 4–10. Proper storage of lead aprons. *A*, Lead apron hung on an appropriately designed hanger by loops at the shoulder region. *B*, Lead apron hung on an appropriately designed hanger by loops at the bottom edge of the apron.

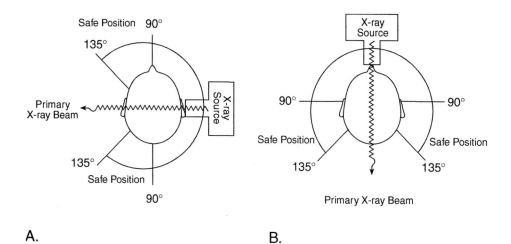

Figure 4–11. The safest operator locations to avoid exposure from the primary beam of radiation are between 90° and 135° to the path of the primary beam. Operators should avoid being located on the same side of the patient as the x-ray source and should never stand in the path of the primary beam. *A*, X-ray source lateral to the patient. *B*, X-ray source anterior to the patient.

instructed in the proper way to stabilize the film in the patient's mouth. Handicapped individuals may require sedation or other alternatives to elicit cooperation. Use of the fastest image receptor available will allow for a shorter exposure time and minimize the loss of image sharpness caused by patient motion.

The potential exists for radiation to leak from the machine tubehead during exposures. Operators should never hold the x-ray machine tubehead during an exposure. The suspension arm and its yoke around the tubehead should be adjusted so that the tubehead remains stable once positioned for an exposure.

Exposure of office staff to occupational radiation can be monitored using film badges supplied by commercial services. Film badges are returned to the monitoring service at regular intervals throughout the year, and a report of individual employee exposure levels is supplied to the subscriber shortly thereafter. Staff members supplied with radiation monitoring devices are cautioned not to leave the badge inadvertently near an x-ray unit during business hours. As exposures are made with the nearby machine, the film inside the monitoring badge will be exposed to the radiation, and an erroneously high-dose reading will be given in the next report. A single staff person should be assigned the duty of monitoring office-wide compliance in wearing the monitoring device daily and in regular submission of the badges to the monitoring service. The dentist should be responsible for evaluation of the monitoring reports.

Quality Assurance

A written quality assurance (QA) program will help ensure that a facility will consistently produce radiographic images of high quality at minimal cost and the lowest dose possible to patients and office personnel.

A comprehensive QA program entails the regular testing of all equipment for proper function and monitoring of all procedures for consistency. In addition to the tests performed annually on x-ray machines, the darkroom and film-processing equipment and procedures must be monitored on a daily or weekly basis. Consistent monitoring will guard against an incipient loss of image quality over the effective life span of the processing solutions.

The main purpose of a comprehensive QA program is the reduction of patient dose by minimizing the need to retake radiographs owing to loss of image quality caused by an equipment malfunction. In addition, fewer repeat radiographs result in a savings of time and expense for both patients and practitioners. Routine and scheduled testing and maintenance procedures also make it easier for facilities to comply with state and federal regulations regarding the operation of equipment for the generation of ionizing radiation.

RISK FROM DIAGNOSTIC IMAGING WITH NONIONIZING RADIATION

Ultrasound Imaging

Research has not demonstrated any negative effects from the use of ultrasound energy in diagnostic image production. In vitro and animal studies have produced negative sequelae when the applied ultrasound energy was far in excess of that used in diagnostic applications. These negative effects include free radical formation, elevation of tissue temperature, cavitation, and the creation of viscous stress.

Cavitation is described as the formation of tiny gas bubbles or cavities within the fluid components of cellular structures. Temperature elevation and cavitation may cause structural changes in biomolecules and free radical formation, as well as disrupt membranes. The rate of biochemical reactions may also be affected by elevated tissue temperatures. Viscous stress results when fluids of different viscosities residing on opposite sides of a membrane are subjected to ultrasound energy. The result is that these fluids begin to stream across the membrane, and this "microstreaming" has the potential to disrupt the membrane.

Magnetic Resonance Imaging

As in ultrasound imaging, no negative effects have been demonstrated from magnetic resonance technology applied to diagnostic imaging. Excessive levels of the energy types used in MRI applied to living systems in a research environment have resulted in negative effects. Deleterious effects can result from exposure to an excessively strong external magnetic field, from an external magnetic field varying in its strength or direction, and from radiofrequency pulses. The main effect of the radiofrequency energy is tissue temperature elevation.

Subjecting a living organism to a strong external magnetic field may initiate changes in membrane permeability, enzyme kinetics, neural conduction, and muscle activity. Intentional variation of the properties of an external magnetic field may have an effect on bone remodeling and cardiac muscle activity.

Although no predictable damage has been demonstrated for either ultrasound or magnetic resonance imaging, the benefits to be gained from the results of the test must outweigh the possible risk of subjecting the patient to the procedure.

DESIGN FEATURES OF A RADIATION-SAFE DENTAL FACILITY

Compliance with the occupational and nonoccupational dose limits of the persons occupying a facility during business hours dictates the features of office design for radiation safety. Potential radiation exposure of each of the following areas must be considered: the reception area, private and business offices, restrooms, staff lounge, laboratory, and consultation room and operatories. If the dental facility is directly adjacent to other businesses or offices, these areas must also be addressed. The primary features of office design are the location of each x-ray machine and the directions in which it is capable of projecting its primary x-ray beam. In addition to the source of radiation, the following factors must also be considered: protective barriers, workload, kilovoltage peak, distance, radiation status, and occupancy factors.

Sources of Radiation

Each x-ray machine tubehead presents three sources of radiation from which office occupants must be protected. The first and most significant source is the x-ray beam exiting from the end of the collimator (PID), the *primary beam* of radiation. The second source is *secondary radiation* composed principally of scatter radiation from the patient's face. The third source is *leakage radiation* from the tubehead housing while x rays are being generated.

Protective Barriers and Related Factors

Appropriate barriers must be in place between the source of radiation and the individuals in the facility. Barriers are classified as *primary* and *secondary*. Barriers designed to be in the path of the primary beam are primary barriers. The most common primary barriers are the operatory walls behind and on either side of the patient. Secondary barriers are intended to absorb radiation such as that scattered from the patient and the leakage from the tubehead. Typical secondary barriers are the ceiling and floor.

Barrier specifications for each operatory will depend on the following five elements: the *total workload* of the x-ray machine in each operatory, the *maximum kVp* at which the x-ray machine will be operated, the *distance* from the x-ray source to the people occupying the facility, the *radiation status* of the people in the facility, and the *occupancy factor* for all areas immediately adjacent to the operatory housing the x-ray unit.

Total workload is determined for each x-ray machine in the facility, and this includes the values for intraoral and extraoral projections if the particular machine is used for both purposes. Workload is recorded as units of mAs and thus is related to beam intensity for the unit being evaluated. The intraoral workload is calculated by multiplying the mAs used to produce a diagnostic quality periapical radiograph of a maxillary first molar times the average number of intraoral films exposed by the unit per week. The extraoral workload is determined similarly by multiplying the mAs used to generate a diagnostic quality image of the extraoral projection under consideration by the number of films exposed by the unit in a week. This calculation is performed for each type of extraoral projection taken in the particular operatory. The sum of the individual workloads is the total workload for that x-ray machine.

The penetrating ability or quality of the x-ray beam is determined by the kilovoltage peak (kVp) setting on the x-ray machine control box. This design feature is relevant to protecting areas adjacent to the x-ray operatory that are in the path of the primary beam of radiation. This factor is recorded as the highest kVp setting used for that machine. Barrier thickness and effectiveness requirements increase as the maximum kVp setting becomes greater.

The inverse square law is applied when determining a safe distance and barrier requirements for the source of radiation from office occupants. The greater the distance from the radiation source, the thinner the barrier can be. Recall that as the distance from the source of radiation is doubled, the intensity of the incident radiation will be reduced to one fourth of its original intensity.

The radiation status of individuals relates to whether they are occupational or nonoccupational persons. At any given time an office population usually will include both types of individuals. Recall that the maximum permissible dose (MPD) for pregnant occupational workers and the nonoccupational general population is one tenth the MPD of occupational workers in general. Compliance with optimal barrier requirements necessitates barrier thickness and efficiency adequate to protect pregnant employees and the nonoccupational population throughout the office.

The occupancy factor refers to the frequency with which an area or room adjacent to an operatory that houses an x-ray machine is occupied. All areas in a dental office are assigned an occupancy factor value of 1.

The information collected by applying these five factors to a facility is used in conjunction with several tables in the *NCRP Handbook Number 35* to convert the data into the appropriate thickness for the material being considered as the barrier. Barrier thickness and efficiency vary in terms of equivalent millimeters of lead or inches of concrete or other materials. A typical dental office will have a relatively low workload, and several layers of common building materials, such as drywall, can be used to provide the appropriate equivalent of a lead or concrete barrier.

HAZARDOUS WASTE IN RADIOGRAPHY

The potentially hazardous materials associated with radiographic procedures are the x-ray developer and fixer solutions and their by-products, and the lead foil from intraoral film packets. All office personnel must be familiar with the proper methods of the handling and disposal of these materials.

Material Safety Data Sheet

All potentially hazardous materials, regardless of their application, must be accompanied by a *Material Safety Data Sheet* (MSDS) when delivered by the vendor. The Occupational Safety and Health Administration (OSHA) requires that employers make the MSDS for each material used in the office readily available to all employees. The MSDS presents information about the manufacturer of the product; the hazardous ingredients in the product and their identity; the physical and chemical properties of the material, along with its fire, explosion, and reactivity potential; and precautions to be taken for the safe handling, use, and control of accidental spills of the material.

A single person should be appointed as the hazardous materials coordinator for the office. All personnel should be familiar with the materials in the facility for which an MSDS exists, in the event of an emergency involving any of these substances. The dentist, or person responsible for the facility and its employees, is charged by OSHA with the duty of providing mandatory education for the entire office staff in the identification, proper handling, and disposal of materials accompanied by an MSDS.

The United States Department of Labor provides a generic MSDS, but manufacturers are permitted to present the essential data in a format that is the most concise for their product.

Handling Radiographic Chemicals and Waste

Radiograph-processing chemicals and the lead foil from intraoral film packets require proper handling and disposal. The developer is a weak acid solution and the fixer a basic solution, each of which could be a health or an environmental hazard. The darkroom should be well ventilated to prevent excessive breathing of the fumes from the processing solutions. Office staff who are responsible for processing-equipment operation and maintenance and for the solutions used in the equipment must be educated regarding the hazards involved. OSHA has established standards for personal protective equipment (PPE), which include wearing the appropriate type of gloves for hand protection, the appropriate mask for face and mucous membrane protection, protective safety goggles to cover the eyes, and protective clothing to guard against the skin being exposed to certain hazardous materials.

Federal OSHA standards state that employers, including dentists, must conduct an assessment of hazards in the workplace (excluding bloodborne pathogens) and select personal protective equipment that will protect employees from any of the hazards found; train employees in the proper selection and use of PPE; and certify in writing that the hazard assessment has been completed and that employees have received the required training.

Disposal of Radiographic Waste

The chemical nature of the processing solutions, one being a base and the other an acid, allows exhausted solutions of each to be mixed to create a neutral solution. This neutralized solution still represents a health and environmental hazard if not properly disposed of. In some locations it is not acceptable to rinse this mixture down the drain or to flush it down the toilet. It is recommended that dental offices collect exhausted processing solutions and use licensed waste disposal companies specializing in hazardous waste pick-up and disposal.

A major contaminant of exhausted fixer solution is dissolved silver. The silver can be recovered from the solution by a chemical or an electroplating method and sold to reclamation or refining companies as scrap silver.

The lead foil in intraoral film packets is also a health and environmental concern. A simple solution to this problem is to collect the lead foil as it is separated from the exposed film packet and sell it to a scrap metal dealer when a sufficient quantity has accumulated. Chapter 7 also provides information about management of waste from dental radiography.

REFERENCES

Atchison KA: Guidelines for prescribing dental radiographs. In Goaz PW, White SC: Oral Radiology: Principles and Interpretation, 3rd edition, p 24. St. Louis, CV Mosby, 1994.

Baum BJ, Bodner L, Fox PC, et al: Therapy-induced dysfunction of salivary glands: Implications for oral health. Spec Care Dent 1985;5:274–277.

Biological Effects of Ionizing Radiation report. III: The effects on populations of exposure to low levels of ionizing radiation. Washington, DC, National Academy Press, 1980.

Biological Effects of Ionizing Radiation report. V: Health effects of exposure to low levels of ionizing radiation. Washington, DC, National Academy Press, 1990.

Brooks SL: A study of selection criteria for intraoral dental radiography. Oral Surg Oral Med Oral Pathol 1986;62:234–239.

Bushong SC: Concepts of radiation. In Radiologic Science for Technologists: Physics, Biology, and Protection, 4th edition, p 1. St. Louis, CV Mosby, 1988.

Bushong SC: Fundamentals of physics. In Radiologic Science for Technologists: Physics, Biology, and Protection, 4th edition, p 15. St. Louis, CV Mosby, 1988.

Bushong SC: The atom. In Radiologic Science for Technologists: Physics, Biology, and Protection, 4th edition, p 30. St. Louis, CV Mosby, 1988.

Bushong SC: Beam-restricting devices. In Radiologic Science for Technologists: Physics, Biology, and Protection, 4th edition, p 182. St. Louis, CV Mosby, 1988.

Bushong SC: Design of radiologic imaging facilities. In Radiologic Science for Technologists: Physics, Biology, and Protection, 4th edition, p 443. St. Louis, CV Mosby, 1988.

Bushong SC: Fundamental principles of radiobiology. In Radiologic Science for Technologists: Physics, Biology, and Protection, 4th edition, p 455. St. Louis, CV Mosby, 1988.

Bushong SC: Molecular and cellular radiobiology. In Radiologic Science for Technologists: Physics, Biology, and Protection, 4th edition, p 477. St. Louis, CV Mosby, 1988.

Bushong SC: Early effects of radiation. In Radiologic Science for Technologists: Physics, Biology, and Protection, 4th edition, p 495. St. Louis, CV Mosby, 1988.

Bushong SC: Late effects of radiation. In Radiologic Science for Technologists: Physics, Biology, and Protection, 4th edition, p 513. St. Louis, CV Mosby, 1988.

Bushong SC: Health physics. In Radiologic Science for Technologists: Physics, Biology, and Protection, 4th edition, p 535. St. Louis, CV Mosby, 1988.

Bushong SC: Designing for radiation protection. In Radiologic Science for Technologists: Physics, Biology, and Protection, 4th edition, p 552. St. Louis, CV Mosby, 1988.

Bushong SC: Radiation protection procedures. In Radiologic Science for Technologists: Physics, Biology, and Protection, 4th edition, p 571. St. Louis, CV Mosby, 1988.

Bushong SC: Physical principles of diagnostic ultrasound. In Radiologic Science for Technologists: Physics, Biology, and Protection, 4th edition, p 595. St. Louis, CV Mosby, 1988.

Bushong SC: Diagnostic ultrasound instrumentation and operation. In Radiologic Science for Technologists: Physics, Biology, and Protection, 4th edition, p 614. St. Louis, CV Mosby, 1988.

Committee on the Biological Effects of Ionizing Radiation: Health effects of exposure to low levels of ionizing radiation. In Biological Effects of Ionizing Radiation report. V. Washington, DC, National Academy Press, 1990.

Frederiksen NL: In Goaz PW, White SC: Oral Radiology: Principles and Interpretation, 3rd edition, p 47. St. Louis, CV Mosby, 1994.

Fromm M, Littman P, Raney RB, et al: Late effects after treatment of twenty children with soft tissue sarcomas of the head and neck. Cancer 1986;57:2070–2076.

Gibbs SJ: Influence of organs in the ICRP's remainder on effective dose equivalent computed for diagnostic radiation exposures. Health Physics 1989;56:515–520.

Gibbs SJ, Pujol A, Chen TS, et al: Patient risk from intraoral dental radiography. Dentomaxillofac Radiol 1988;17:15–23.

Goaz PW, White SC: Biologic effects of radiation. In Oral Radiology: Principles and Interpretation, 3rd edition, p 24. St. Louis, CV Mosby, 1994.

Hall EJ: The physics and chemistry of radiation absorption. In Radiobiology for the Radiologist, 3rd edition, p 1. Philadelphia, JB Lippincott, 1988.

Hall EJ: Dose-response relationships for normal tissues. In Radiobiology for the Radiologist, 3rd edition, p 39. Philadelphia, JB Lippincott, 1988.

Hall EJ: Radiosensitivity and cell age in the mitotic cycle. In Radiobiology for the Radiologist, 3rd edition, p 91. Philadelphia, JB Lippincott, 1988.

Hall EJ: Radiation damage and the dose-rate effect. In Radiobiology for the Radiologist, 3rd edition, p 107. Philadelphia, JB Lippincott, 1988.

Hall EJ: The oxygen effect and reoxygenation. In Radiobiology for the Radiologist, 3rd edition, p 137. Philadelphia, JB Lippincott, 1988.

Hall EJ: LET and RBE. In Radiobiology for the Radiologist, 3rd edition, p 161. Philadelphia, JB Lippincott, 1988.

Hall EJ: Radiosensitizers. In Radiobiology for the Radiologist, 3rd edition, p 179. Philadelphia, JB Lippincott, 1988.

Hall EJ: Radioprotectors. In Radiobiology for the Radiologist, 3rd edition, p 201. Philadelphia, JB Lippincott, 1988.

Hall EJ: Time, dose, and fractionation in radiotherapy. In Radiobiology for the Radiologist, 3rd edition, p 239. Philadelphia, JB Lippincott, 1988.

Hall EJ: Sensitivity of tissues. In Radiobiology for the Radiologist, 3rd edition, p 357. Philadelphia, JB Lippincott, 1988.

Hall EJ: Acute effects of whole-body irradiation. In Radiobiology for the Radiologist, 3rd edition, p 365. Philadelphia, JB Lippincott, 1988.

Hall EJ: Late effects of radiation: Carcinogenesis and nonspecific life shortening. In Radiobiology for the Radiologist, 3rd edition, p 385. Philadelphia, JB Lippincott, 1988.

Hall EJ: Late effects of radiation: Genetic changes. In Radiobiology for the Radiologist, 3rd edition, p 412. Philadelphia, JB Lippincott, 1988.

Hall EJ: Effects of radiation on the embryo and fetus. In Radiobiology for the Radiologist, 3rd edition, p 445. Philadelphia, JB Lippincott, 1988.

Hall EJ: Diagnostic radiology and nuclear medicine: Risk versus benefit. In Radiobiology for the Radiologist, 3rd edition, p 467. Philadelphia, JB Lippincott, 1988.

Hall EJ: Radiation protection. In Radiobiology for the Radiologist, 3rd edition, p 505. Philadelphia, JB Lippincott, 1988.

Hollender L: Decision making in radiographic imaging. J Dent Educ 1992;56(12):834–843.

Leavitt DD, Schiager KJ: Environmental issues in radiology. Invest Radiol 1990;25:942–956.

Maulik D: Biologic effects of ultrasound. Clin Obstet Gynecol 1989;32:645–659.

Mettler FA, Moseley RD: Basic radiation physics, chemistry, and biology. In Medical Effects of Ionizing Radiation, p 1. Orlando, Florida, Grune and Stratton, 1985.

Mettler FA, Moseley RD: Sources of radiation exposure. In Medical Effects of Ionizing Radiation, p 31. Orlando, Florida, Grune and Stratton, 1985.

Mettler FA, Moseley RD: Effects on genetic material. In Medical Effects of Ionizing Radiation, p 54. Orlando, Florida, Grune and Stratton, 1985.

Mettler FA, Moseley RD: Cancer induction and dose-response models. In Medical Effects of Ionizing Radiation, p 74. Orlando, Florida, Grune and Stratton, 1985.

Mettler FA, Moseley RD: Direct effects of radiation. In Medical Effects of Ionizing Radiation, p 126. Orlando, Florida, Grune and Stratton, 1985.

Mettler FA, Moseley RD: Radiation exposure in-utero. In Medical Effects of Ionizing Radiation, p 202. Orlando, Florida, Grune and Stratton, 1985.

National Center for Health Care Technology: Dental radiology: A summary of recommendations from the Technology Assessment Forum. J Am Dent Assoc 1981;103:423–425.

National Council on Radiation Protection and Measurements (NCRP): Medical radiation exposure of pregnant and potentially pregnant women. Report 54. Washington, DC, NCRP Publications, 1977.

1990 Recommendations. International Commission on Radiological Protection: ICRP Publication 60, Annals of the ICRP 21, New York, 1990.

Preston-Martin S, Thomas CC, White SC, et al: Prior exposure to medical and dental x rays related to tumors of the parotid gland. J Natl Cancer Inst 1988;80:943–949.

Preston-Martin S, White SC: Brain and salivary gland tumors related to prior dental radiography: Implications for current practice. J Am Dent Assoc 1990;120:151–158.

Pyykomen H, Malmstrom M, Oikarinen VJ, et al: Late effects of radiation treatment of tongue and floor-of-mouth cancer on the dentition, saliva secretion, mucous membranes and the lower jaw. Int J Oral Maxillofac Surg 1986;15:401–409.

Razmus TF: Radiation biology. In Miles DA, Van Dis ML, Razmus TF: Basic Principles of Oral and Maxillofacial Radiology, p 21. Philadelphia, WB Saunders, 1992.

Razmus TF: Radiation protection. In Miles DA, Van Dis ML, Razmus TF: Basic Principles of Oral and Maxillofacial Radiology, p 37. Philadelphia, WB Saunders, 1992.

Rothwell BR: Prevention and treatment of the orofacial complications of radiotherapy. J Am Dent Assoc 1987;114:316–322.

Underhill TE, Chilvarquer I, Kimura K, et al: Radiobiological risk estimation from dental radiology. I, Absorbed dose to critical organs. Oral Surg Oral Med Oral Pathol 1988;66:111–120.

Underhill TE, Chilvarquer I, Kimura K, et al: Radiobiological risk estimation from dental radiology. II, Cancer incidence and fatality. Oral Surg Oral Med Oral Pathol 1988;66:261–267.

U.S. Department of Health and Human Services: The selection of patients for x-ray examinations. Washington, DC, HHS Publ (FDA) 88-8273, 1987.

U.S. Department of Labor, Occupational Safety and Health Administration: Material Safety Data Sheet. Form approved OMB No. 1218-0072. Washington, DC, 1985.

White SC: 1992 assessment of radiation risks from dental radiology. Dentomaxillofac Radiol 1992;21:118–126.

5

INTRAORAL RADIOGRAPHIC TECHNIQUES

GAIL F. WILLIAMSON

Intraoral Image Receptors

Periapical Image Production

Bitewing Image Production

Occlusal Image Production

Common Intraoral Technical Errors and Artifacts

Difficult Clinical Receptor Placement Situations

Localization Techniques

INTRAORAL IMAGE RECEPTORS

Intraoral image receptors include various sizes of radiographic film and direct digital imaging sensors that are placed inside the mouth to record the teeth and bony structures of the oral cavity. The x-ray source is aligned externally over the receptor site, often with the aid of a receptor holder that has an extraoral beam alignment guide. Upon exposure, the x-ray beam penetrates the structures and produces a latent image (pattern of the structures) on the receptor. The visible image is the result of chemical or computer processing of the latent image. There are three basic types of intraoral radiographs: periapical, bitewing, and occlusal. Some direct digital imaging receptors are available in three sizes for periapical and bitewing image applications. The sensor size itself and the range of available sensor sizes vary among the manufacturers of direct digital imaging systems.

Periapical Images

A periapical image records an entire tooth or a group of teeth as well as the surrounding supporting structures: trabecular bone, lamina dura, and

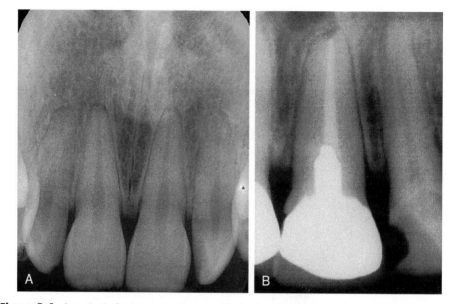

Figure 5–1. A periapical image records an entire tooth or group of teeth as well as the surrounding supporting structures. *A,* A periapical radiograph of the maxillary central incisor teeth. *B,* A direct digital image (DDI) of an endodontically treated maxillary left central incisor.

periodontal ligament space (Fig. 5–1). A diagnostic periapical image depicts the area of interest, including the entire length of the teeth from the crowns to the root apices, the interproximal surfaces of the teeth, and at least 3 to 4 mm of bone surrounding the root apices. Periapical images are used to determine tooth morphology and abnormalities of the teeth or supporting structures, such as caries, periodontal disease, and periapical pathosis. Selected periapical images may be taken to record specific teeth, or a complete series of periapical images may be taken to record the entire dentition.

Periapical radiographic film is available in several sizes: 2, 1, and 0 (Fig. 5–2). Size 2 (31 × 41 mm) film is the universal size for adult periapical imaging. The exposure side of the film is the plain white side of the packet earmarked by the film identification dot convexity (Fig. 5–3). Typically, the film receptor is positioned vertically for anterior views and horizontally for

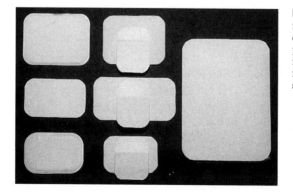

Figure 5–2. The various intraoral film sizes are pictured here. The left column includes the sizes 2, 1, and 0 periapical film. The middle column includes the sizes 2, 3, and 0 bitewing film. The right column displays the size 4 occlusal film.

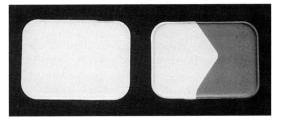

Figure 5–3. The exposure side of the film packet is the plain white side; the nonexposure side of the film packet is the two-color side.

posterior views, with the film identification dot oriented toward the coronal aspect of the image. Size 1 (24 × 40 mm) film is frequently used instead of size 2 film for adult anterior periapical imaging because its width dimension permits better placement in the anterior segment of the arches. In addition, the size 1 film receptor is useful for periapical imaging of the mixed dentition. Size 0 (22 × 35 mm) film is used primarily for periapical imaging of the primary or mixed dentition to accommodate the size of the child patient's oral cavity.

Some direct digital sensors (Fig. 5–4) are available in several sizes that are comparable to sizes 2, 1, and 0 film (the exact height, width, and thickness vary among manufacturers). Currently, the most common direct digital sensor size is comparable to the size 1 periapical film and is placed vertically in both the anterior and posterior regions of the mouth. Direct digital imaging x-ray sensors are thicker (6.0 to 11.7 mm) and more rigid than intraoral film packets. Usually, the level, noncontoured surface of the sensor is the exposure side. In addition, these sensors are attached to a cable that transmits the latent image data to the computer to produce the visible image. The operator should exercise care in positioning the sensor so that the cable is not bent or damaged by the biting forces of the teeth.

A typical film-based periapical survey of the adult dentition consists of 14 to 16 periapical views. Periapical surveys may consist of all size 2 images or, often, a combination of size 1 images in the anterior regions and size 2 images in the posterior regions. Direct digital imaging periapical surveys vary in number from 14 to 20 views, depending upon the size of the receptor used for image acquisition.

Figure 5–4. Direct digital imaging (DDI) sensors come in a variety of sizes. The vertical sensor on the left is 22 × 41 × 8 mm, comparable to the size 1 film (Sens-A-Ray, Regam Medical Systems, Sundsvall, Sweden). The top right sensor is 28 × 43 × 6 mm, comparable to the size 2 film (Computed Dental Radiography, Schick Technologies, Inc., Long Island City, New York). The bottom right sensor is 24.2 × 37.5 × 11.7 mm, and is comparable to the size 1 film (RadioVisioGraphy, Trophy Radiologie, Paris, France).

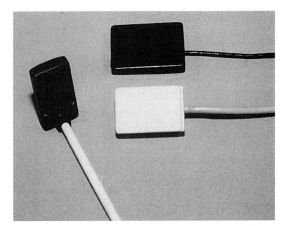

Bitewing Images

A bitewing image displays the crowns, interproximal surfaces, and inter-dental alveolar bone of both the maxillary and the mandibular teeth (Fig. 5–5). A diagnostic bitewing image depicts the area of interest, including the interproximal surfaces of the maxillary and mandibular crowns and the alveolar crestal bone. Typically, these images are taken of the posterior teeth and are used to determine interproximal caries, defective restorations, and alveolar crestal bone height. These images can be taken in the anterior region as well and may be positioned in either the horizontal or vertical dimension. Frequently, bitewing receptors are placed vertically to record more accurately the alveolar bone height when moderate or advanced periodontal disease is present.

Bitewing radiographic film (see Fig. 5–2) and some direct digital sensors (see Fig. 5–4) are available in several sizes: 2, 1, and 0. The exposure side of the film receptor is the plain white side of the packet earmarked by the film identification dot convexity (see Fig. 5–3), and the level, noncontoured surface of the sensor is the exposure side of the direct digital imaging receptor. Usually, periapical film and sensors can be used for bitewing imaging by applying a bitewing tab or utilizing a bitewing instrument holder to position the receptor. In addition to the aforementioned bitewing film sizes, a size 3 (27 × 54 mm) is available for posterior bitewings (see Fig. 5–2).

The typical adult bitewing survey consists of four size 2 vertically or horizontally placed bitewings; the typical child bitewing survey consists of two horizontally placed bitewings. The receptor size (2, 1, 0) used in the child bitewing survey depends on the child's age, dentition, and size of the oral cavity.

Occlusal Images

An occlusal image records a large portion of the maxilla or mandible that is beyond the scope of a single periapical image (Fig. 5–6). The size 4 (57 × 76 mm) film receptor (see Fig. 5–2) is oriented either in the horizontal or

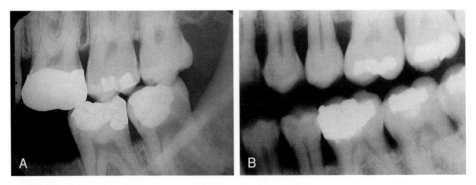

Figure 5–5. A bitewing image displays the crowns, interproximal surfaces, and interdental alveolar bone of both maxillary and mandibular posterior teeth. *A,* Bitewing radiograph. *B,* Direct digital bitewing image.

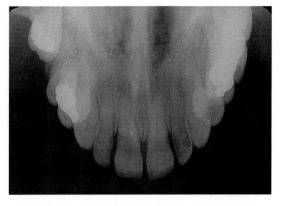

Figure 5-6. An occlusal image records a large portion of the maxilla or mandible that is beyond the scope of a single periapical film. The topographical maxillary anterior occlusal is one example of an occlusal projection.

vertical plane and placed against the occlusal surfaces of the teeth of the arch of interest. The x-ray beam is directed through the desired region with greater angulations than are typically used for periapical radiography. As with other intraoral film receptors, the exposure side of the occlusal film is the plain white side of the packet earmarked by the film identification dot convexity.

There are two types of occlusal projections: topographical and cross-sectional. Topographical projections are frequently used to view a broader area of the maxilla or mandible, impacted teeth, or a large bony lesion, or as a replacement for anterior periapicals in children (size 2 receptors are used for child occlusal radiography) or adults with restricted opening of the mouth. A topographical projection of the anterior maxilla includes the anterior teeth, palate, nasal structures, and maxillary sinus (see Fig. 5–6). The topographical mandibular anterior projection displays the anterior teeth, anterior mandibular bone, and floor of the mouth. Although topographical occlusals are most frequently taken in the anterior regions of the jaws, posterior occlusals of either arch can be taken when indicated. Cross-sectional occlusals are most typically used to localize objects such as supernumerary teeth, impacted teeth, foreign objects, and salivary stones in the sublingual and submandibular glands, or to determine mediolateral expansion of the jaws or the displacement of fractures of the maxilla and mandible.

Surveys

The type and number of radiographic images needed to survey each patient's oral condition are determined on an individual basis using selection criteria guidelines. The prescribed survey will vary among individuals; some patients will require bitewings, others may require selected periapicals of specific teeth, whereas still others may require a combination of selected periapicals and bitewings or a full mouth survey. A complete or full mouth survey consists of 14 to 16 periapical views and two to four posterior bitewing views (Fig. 5–7).

PERIAPICAL IMAGE PRODUCTION

Four basic technical rules govern accurate image formation:

1. The receptor should be placed parallel to the structures to be imaged.

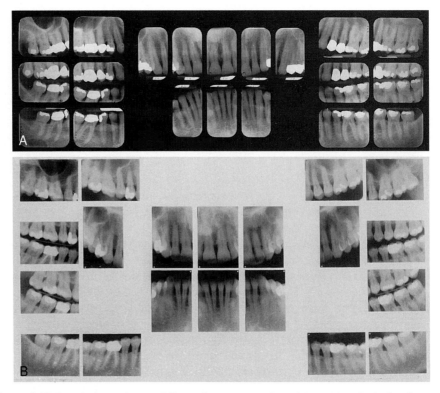

Figure 5–7. A typical complete or full-mouth survey consists of 14 to 16 periapical and two to four bitewing views. *A,* Full-mouth radiographic survey with both size 1 and size 2 films. *B,* A DDI full-mouth survey with size 2 sensor images.

2. The receptor should be placed as close to the structures to be imaged as practical (object-receptor distance).

3. The central ray (center of the x-ray beam) should be placed perpendicular (at a right angle) to the object and receptor.

4. The longest source (focal)-to-receptor distance (PID* length) as practical should be used.

The purpose of these guidelines is to minimize the geometric characteristics of unsharpness, magnification, and shape distortion that are present to some degree in every radiographic image. To visualize how these rules influence image formation, the reader can apply the same rules to casting the shadow of an object onto a wall with a flashlight. Alteration of the rules affects the outline sharpness, overall size, and shape of the shadow cast on the wall. X-ray produced images behave in a similar manner and will display the same types of image distortion.

There are two basic techniques for producing film-based or direct digital periapical imaging: the paralleling technique and the bisecting angle technique. Both are based on a particular relationship between the object and receptor, which determines the resultant angulation of the x-ray source. The

---

*PID, position indicating device.

paralleling technique conforms to most of the rules for accurate image formation and is the preferred technique for intraoral imaging because of its image accuracy and superior representation of the teeth and surrounding structures. The bisecting angle technique conforms to only one of the rules of accurate image formation and, therefore, should be considered an adjunct or supplemental technique. No matter how well executed, the bisecting angle technique produces image shape distortion. However, it can be employed in difficult or atypical clinical situations in which the paralleling technique is not possible. The bisecting angle technique is discussed later in the chapter.

PARALLELING TECHNIQUE

The paralleling technique requires the receptor to be placed both vertically and horizontally parallel to the long axes of the teeth to be imaged and the x-ray beam to be directed at right angles (perpendicular) to both the teeth and the image receptor (Fig. 5–8). This relationship of the teeth, receptor, and x-ray beam minimizes geometric distortion. To achieve parallelism between the long axes of the teeth and the receptor, the clinician should move the receptor lingual to the teeth to secure the final placement. In doing so, the object-to-receptor distance is increased and results in image magnification and geometric blurriness. To compensate for this, a long source-to-receptor distance, or 16-inch PID, should be used. This reduces the magnification and geometric blurriness, producing an image with increased definition.

Paralleling Instruments

A film holder must be used to position the receptor parallel to the structures to be imaged. Receptor holders with extraoral PID alignment guides are

Figure 5–8. The paralleling technique requires the receptor to be placed both vertically and horizontally parallel to the long axis of the tooth to be imaged. The x-ray beam is centered and directed at right angles to both the tooth and the receptor. The central ray is designated as CR.

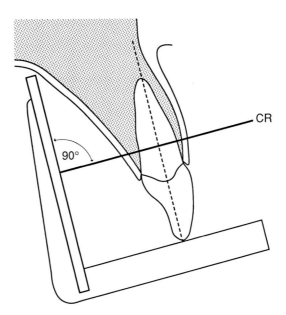

available for both film-based paralleling technique (Fig. 5–9) and direct digital imaging paralleling technique (Fig. 5–10). When assembled correctly and used according to paralleling technique guidelines, these holders can assist the clinician in producing consistent diagnostic images with a minimum of technical errors. Another option is to use a standard biteblock to maintain the film position. The clinician must pay strict attention to paralleling technique parameters in order to produce a quality image in this manner.

X-Ray Beam Angulation and Alignment

The x-ray beam should be aligned so that the vertical and horizontal angulations are directed perpendicular to the long axes of the teeth and the receptor. In addition, the center of the x-ray beam (central ray) should be positioned over the center of the image receptor (see Fig. 5–8).

The vertical angulation of the x-ray beam can be adjusted by moving the PID up or down according to a scale on the side of the x-ray tube head. Positive vertical angles are formed when the PID is directed down toward the floor, whereas negative vertical angles are formed when the PID is directed up toward the ceiling. Generally speaking, positive vertical angulations are used with maxillary periapical placements and negative vertical angulations are used with mandibular periapical placements. The vertical angulation controls the long axis dimension or length of the recorded image. Errors in vertical angle either lengthen or shorten the long axis size of the image.

The horizontal angulation of the x-ray beam is adjusted by moving the PID right or left in the horizontal plane. This angulation is determined relative to the horizontal plane of both the teeth and the receptor. The horizontal angulation should direct the x-ray beam through the interproximal surfaces of the teeth, which places the beam perpendicular to the horizontal planes of the teeth and receptor. If the horizontal angulation is aligned oblique to the teeth and receptor, overlapping of the proximal surfaces of the teeth occurs, which obscures the visualization of the interproximal areas of the teeth and the alveolar bone crests.

Finally, the x-ray beam must be centered over the receptor to expose the entire surface to the radiation. Misplacement of the central ray results in partial exposure of the receptor and, thus, produces a partial image. The unexposed portion of the partial image is referred to as a "cone cut."

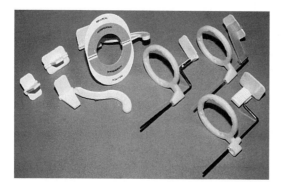

Figure 5–9. A number of paralleling technique instruments with external PID alignment guides are available for film-based imaging. Typical film holders include the VIP2 (Versatile Intraoral Positioner System, UPRAD Corporation, Fort Lauderdale, Florida), located on the left, and the Rinn XCP instruments (Extension Cone Paralleling, Rinn Corporation, Elgin, Illinois), located on the right.

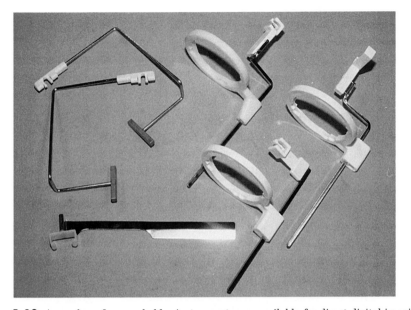

Figure 5-10. A number of sensor holder instruments are available for direct digital imaging. Rinn XCP (Rinn Corporation, Elgin, Illinois) compatible holders, pictured on the right, are available for the CDR sensor (Computed Dental Radiography, Schick Technologies, Inc., Long Island City, New York). RVG sensor holders (Radio VisioGraphy, Trophy Radiologie, Paris, France), top left, are available for either the paralleling or the bisecting angle technique. A Sens-A-Ray (Regam Medical Systems, Sundsvall, Sweden) sensor holder, bottom left, is available for use with the Sens-A-Ray sensor. The biteblock insert is also compatible with the Rinn XCP instruments.

RADIOGRAPHIC PROCEDURAL GUIDELINES

In preparation for the radiographic procedure, a number of preliminary tasks should be completed. The operator properly prepares the x-ray unit and environmental surfaces prior to seating the patient, using effective infection control measures. (A complete discussion of radiographic infection control measures is presented in Chapter 6.) All materials necessary for completion of the radiographic procedures are assembled, such as sterilized receptor holders, the required number of films or the x-ray sensor, cotton rolls, and bitewing tabs.

Patient Seating and Patient Preparation

The patient is seated in an upright but comfortable position. For maxillary periapical and bitewing images, it is recommended that the patient's head be positioned so that the midsagittal plane is perpendicular to the floor and the occlusal plane is parallel to the floor. The patient's head is supported by the headrest. For mandibular exposures, it is helpful to adjust the headrest so that the chin is elevated and the mandibular occlusal plane is parallel to the floor when the patient's mouth is open. These head positions permit easier x-ray beam alignment by the operator. The chair is positioned at a height comfortable for the operator, so that excessive bending or reaching is not required during receptor placement and x-ray beam alignment. Once the patient is properly positioned, the medical history is reviewed with the patient and chart entries made prior to beginning any intraoral procedures.

The patient is instructed to remove any intraoral prostheses, eyeglasses, or metallic objects that may be projected into the x-ray field. These items are safely stored and placed away from the film and instrument working surface. Then the clinician drapes the patient with a lead apron and thyroid collar, taking care to secure them in a comfortable position without obstructing oral structures. The clinician takes time to explain the procedure to the patient and provide instructions to elicit patient cooperation.

Equipment Preparation

The x-ray machine exposure factors are set prior to receptor placement. The patient's physical size is evaluated to determine whether any adjustments in exposure time are necessary prior to beginning the imaging procedures. In addition, the x-ray head is positioned near the area to be imaged for easy operator access.

With direct digital imaging of the patient, some additional preparatory steps are required. The system hardware is readied for the imaging procedures. Effective infection control measures are used to prepare and cover the system hardware (keyboard, mouse, sensor). Some systems have foot control devices to help minimize contact with the computer keyboard and mouse during the imaging procedures. (Refer to Chapter 6 for a complete discussion of direct digital imaging infection control measures.) The system software program has been started using the appropriate prompts, the patient data entered, and the image series format selected prior to beginning the imaging procedures. Then, the operator selects the first image to be acquired on the monitor prior to receptor placement. The hardware, software, and commands vary among direct digital imaging systems. Consult the user's manual for specific system hardware and software operational information.

Receptor Placement Descriptions

The receptor placements described in the following sections are for a 16-image periapical survey. In the film-based periapical survey, size 1 film was used for the anterior periapical views, and size 2 film was used for the posterior periapical views (see Fig. 5–7A). In the direct digital imaging survey, the size 2 sensor was used for both anterior and posterior periapical views (see Fig. 5–7B). The Rinn XCP instrument, a common paralleling technique receptor holder, is shown in Figs. 5–11 to 5–19. Rinn XCP intraoral biteblock components are available for both film and sensor receptors. The receptor placements and x-ray beam alignments are universal among paralleling technique holders.

The patient's oral cavity is examined before beginning the survey. This gives the clinician an opportunity to observe the size of the arches and the arrangement and condition of the teeth and oral tissues, as well as any unusual oral anatomy.

Anterior Receptor Placements

When taking a complete periapical survey, the anterior projections are taken first. Most patients are able to tolerate the anterior placements without difficulty. A size 1 receptor is recommended for imaging the anterior teeth because it permits better and more comfortable placements. Both of these approaches allow the patient to become accustomed to the procedure prior to the posterior receptor placements.

Anterior periapical images include views of the central incisor, lateral incisor, and canine teeth. The receptor is placed vertically with the exposure side of the receptor facing the operator (film dot convexity surface or level, noncontoured sensor surface). For film-based imaging, the dot convexity is oriented toward the coronal aspect of the image. The receptor is centered and placed securely into the instrument biteblock. When the receptor is placed, the mouth is entered with the receptor surface parallel to the incisal edges of the teeth. Then, the apical aspect of the receptor is gently tipped into the palate or floor of the mouth. For mandibular periapical views, the patient is instructed to raise the tongue prior to receptor placement. The receptor is placed lingual to the teeth and the bony ridge. Next, the biteblock is placed against the incisal edges of the teeth to be imaged and the patient instructed to close against the biteblock slowly but gently. Often, a cotton roll placed on the side of the biteblock toward the opposing teeth will help stabilize the receptor placement. The receptor should be vertically and horizontally parallel to the teeth prior to x-ray beam alignment.

The receptor biteblock is a useful placement reference. The biteblock surface should be centered over the incisal edges of the teeth of interest, and the lateral edges of the biteblock should be parallel to the interproximal surfaces of the teeth to be imaged.

Posterior Receptor Placements

Posterior periapical images include views of the distal of the canine, premolar, and molar teeth. Most typically, a size 2 receptor is placed horizontally, with the exposure side of the receptor facing the operator (film dot convexity surface or level, noncontoured sensor surface). For film-based imaging, the dot convexity is oriented toward the coronal aspect of the image. The receptor is centered and placed securely into the instrument biteblock. When placing the receptor, the mouth is entered with the receptor surface parallel to the occlusal surfaces of the posterior teeth. Then, the apical aspect of the receptor is gently tipped into the palate or floor of the mouth. The receptor is placed lingual to the teeth and the bony ridge and toward the midline of the palate on the maxilla or toward the lateral border of the tongue on the mandible. Next, the biteblock is placed against the occlusal surfaces of the teeth to be imaged and the patient instructed to close slowly but gently against the biteblock. Often, a cotton roll placed on the side of the biteblock toward the opposing teeth will help stabilize the receptor placement. The receptor should be vertically and horizontally parallel to the teeth prior to x-ray beam alignment.

The receptor biteblock is a useful placement reference. As in anterior

Text continued on page 142

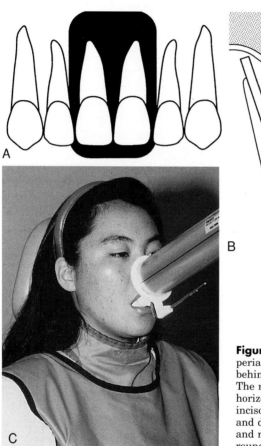

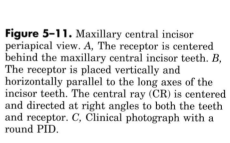

Figure 5–11. Maxillary central incisor periapical view. *A,* The receptor is centered behind the maxillary central incisor teeth. *B,* The receptor is placed vertically and horizontally parallel to the long axes of the incisor teeth. The central ray (CR) is centered and directed at right angles to both the teeth and receptor. *C,* Clinical photograph with a round PID.

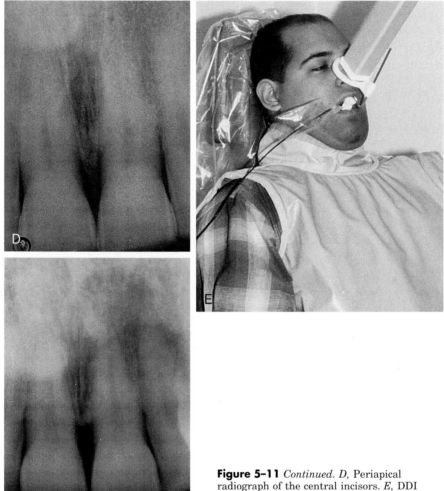

Figure 5–11 *Continued. D,* Periapical radiograph of the central incisors. *E,* DDI clinical photograph with a rectangular PID. *F,* DDI central incisor view.

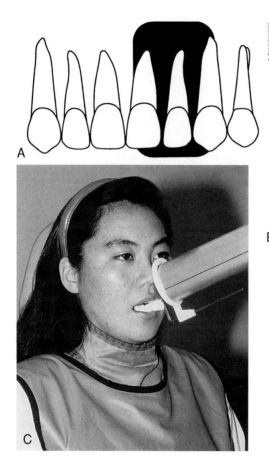

A

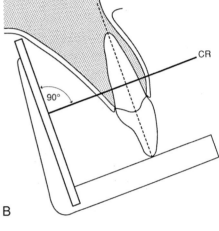

B

C

Figure 5-12. Maxillary lateral incisor periapical view. *A,* The receptor is centered behind the maxillary lateral incisor tooth. *B,* The receptor is placed vertically and horizontally parallel to the long axis of the lateral incisor. The central ray (CR) is centered and directed at right angles to both the teeth and receptor. *C,* Clinical photograph with a round PID.

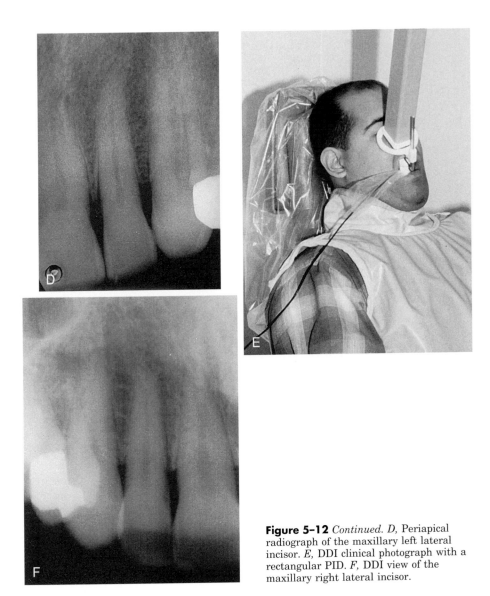

Figure 5–12 *Continued. D,* Periapical radiograph of the maxillary left lateral incisor. *E,* DDI clinical photograph with a rectangular PID. *F,* DDI view of the maxillary right lateral incisor.

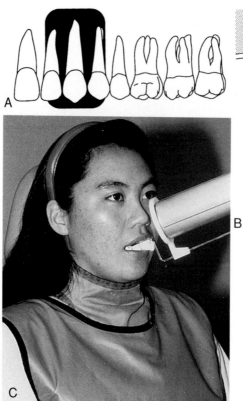

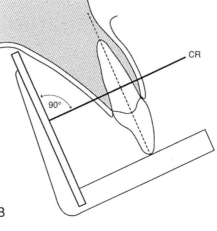

Figure 5–13. Maxillary canine periapical view. *A*, The receptor is centered behind the maxillary canine tooth. *B*, The receptor is placed vertically and horizontally parallel to the long axis of the canine tooth. The central ray (CR) is centered and directed at right angles to both the tooth and receptor. *C*, Clinical photograph with a round PID.

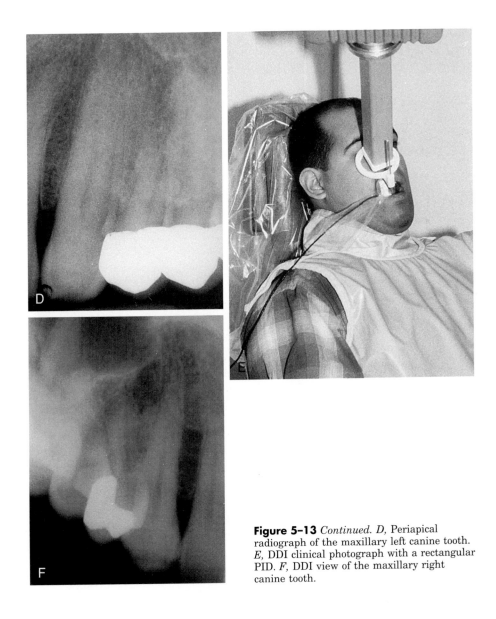

Figure 5–13 *Continued. D,* Periapical radiograph of the maxillary left canine tooth. *E,* DDI clinical photograph with a rectangular PID. *F,* DDI view of the maxillary right canine tooth.

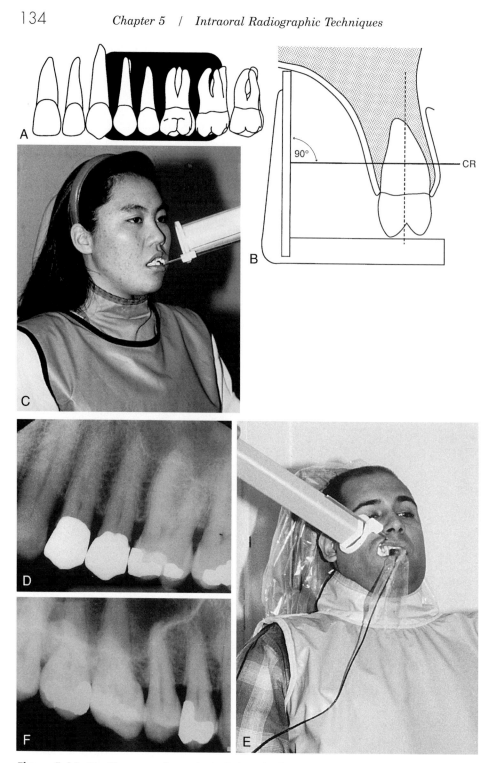

Figure 5-14. Maxillary premolar periapical view. *A,* The receptor is centered behind the maxillary canine, premolar, and first molar teeth. *B,* The receptor is placed vertically and horizontally parallel to the long axes of the premolars. The central ray (CR) is centered and directed at right angles to both the teeth and receptor. *C,* Clinical photograph with a round PID. *D,* Periapical radiograph of the maxillary left premolar region. *E,* DDI clinical photograph with a rectangular PID. *F,* DDI view of the maxillary right premolar region.

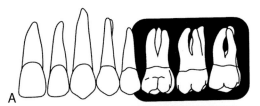

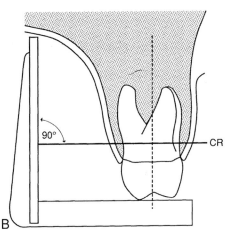

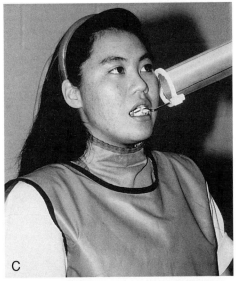

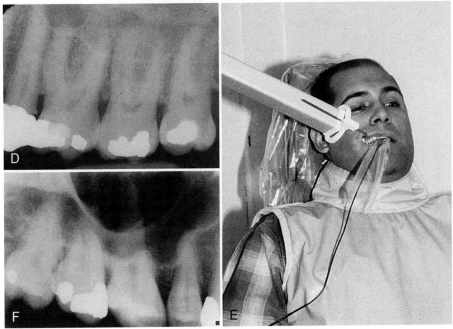

Figure 5–15. Maxillary molar periapical view. *A,* The receptor is centered behind the maxillary molar teeth. *B,* The receptor is placed vertically and horizontally parallel to the long axes of the molars. The central ray (CR) is centered and directed at right angles to both the teeth and receptor. *C,* Clinical photograph with a round PID. *D,* Periapical radiograph of the maxillary left molar region. *E,* DDI clinical photograph with a rectangular PID. *F,* DDI view of the maxillary right molar region.

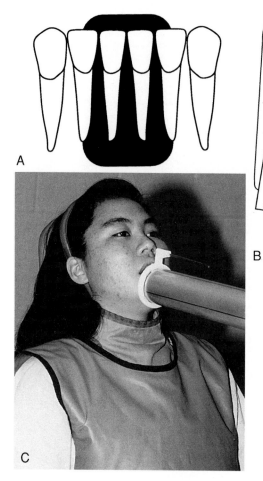

A

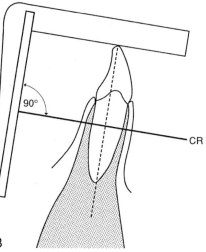

B

C

Figure 5-16. Mandibular incisor periapical view. *A,* The receptor is centered behind the mandibular central incisor teeth. *B,* The receptor is placed vertically and horizontally parallel to the long axes of the central incisors. The central ray (CR) is centered and directed at right angles to both the teeth and receptor. *C,* Clinical photograph with a round PID.

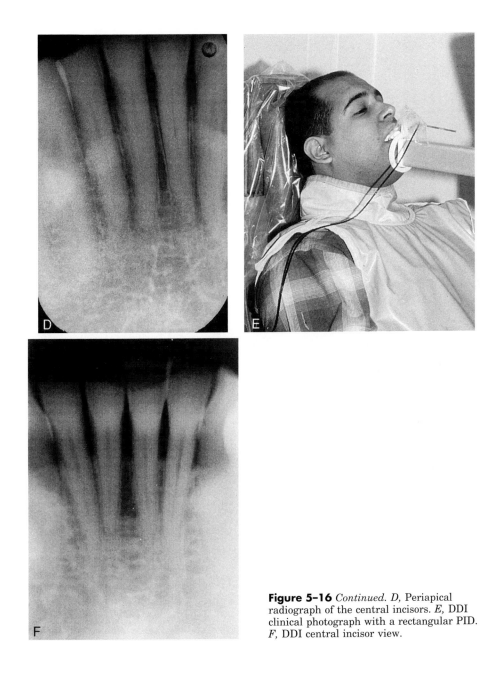

Figure 5–16 *Continued. D*, Periapical radiograph of the central incisors. *E*, DDI clinical photograph with a rectangular PID. *F*, DDI central incisor view.

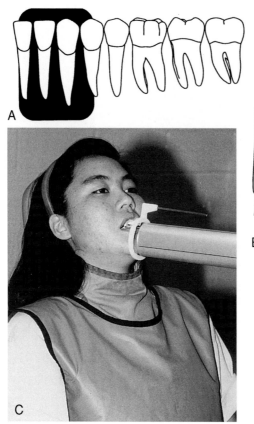

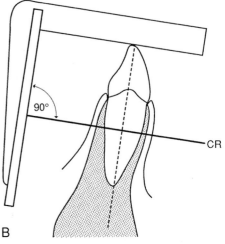

Figure 5-17. Mandibular lateral-canine periapical view. *A,* The receptor is centered behind the mandibular lateral incisor and canine teeth. *B,* The receptor is placed vertically and horizontally parallel to the long axes of the lateral incisor and canine teeth. The central ray (CR) is centered and directed at right angles to both the teeth and receptor. *C,* Clinical photograph with a round PID.

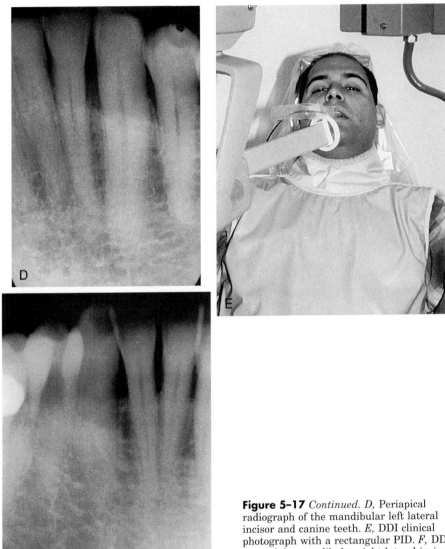

Figure 5-17 *Continued.* *D,* Periapical radiograph of the mandibular left lateral incisor and canine teeth. *E,* DDI clinical photograph with a rectangular PID. *F,* DDI view of the mandibular right lateral incisor and canine teeth.

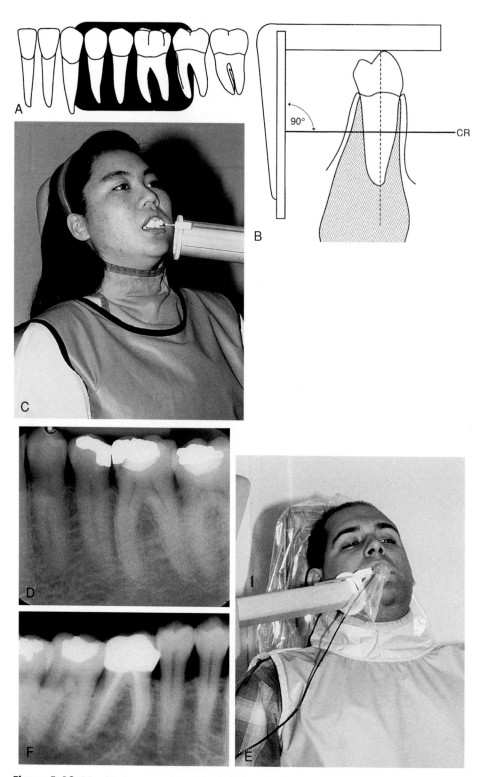

Figure 5–18. Mandibular premolar periapical view. *A,* The receptor is centered behind the mandibular canine, premolar, and first molar teeth. *B,* The receptor is placed vertically and horizontally parallel to the long axes of the premolars. The central ray (CR) is centered and directed at right angles to both the teeth and receptor. *C,* Clinical photograph with a round PID. *D,* Periapical radiograph of the mandibular left premolar region. *E,* DDI clinical photograph with a rectangular PID. *F,* DDI view of the mandibular right premolar region.

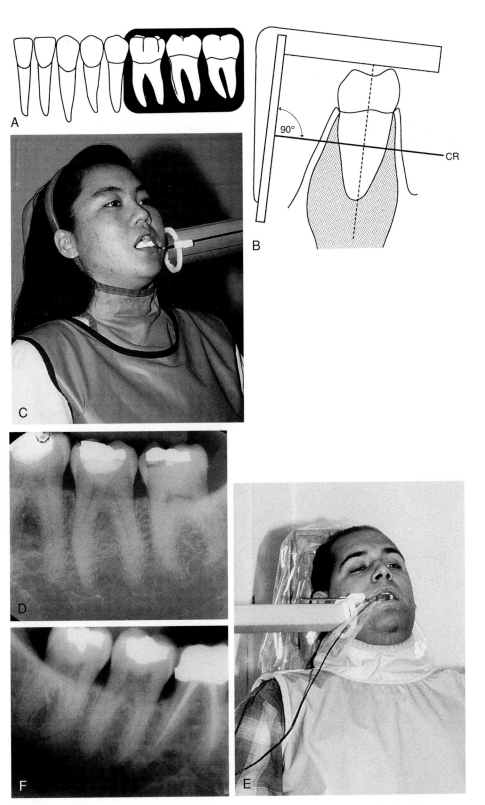

Figure 5-19. Mandibular molar periapical view. *A,* The receptor is centered behind the mandibular molar teeth. *B,* The receptor is placed vertically and horizontally parallel to the long axes of the molars. The central ray (CR) is centered and directed at right angles to both the teeth and receptor. *C,* Clinical photograph with a round PID. *D,* Periapical radiograph of the mandibular left molar region. *E,* DDI clinical photograph with a rectangular PID. *F,* DDI view of the mandibular right molar region.

141

receptor placement, the biteblock surface should be centered over the occlusal surfaces of the teeth of interest and the lateral edges of the biteblock should be parallel to the interproximal surfaces of the teeth to be imaged.

At times, it may be difficult to image the third molar teeth. An additional periapical may be needed to record the third molar in its entirety, especially if it is unerupted or impacted. A useful method for this requires an oblique receptor placement. Rather than placing the receptor horizontally parallel to the teeth, it should be placed 25° to 35° to the horizontal plane. This positions the anterior edge of the receptor near the lingual surface of the first molar crown and the posterior edge rotated toward the midline. The exposure time is increased in order to produce an image of adequate density because of the oblique entry of the x-ray beam. The PID is aligned to the extraoral PID alignment guide, as usual.

BISECTING ANGLE TECHNIQUE

Bisecting angle technique is based on the geometric *Rule of Isometry,* or equilateral triangles. In other words, two triangles will be equal if they share a common side and two equal angles. Applied to imaging, a tooth and its recorded image will be equal in length if they share a common side between them. With bisecting angle periapical technique, the receptor is placed against the lingual surfaces of the teeth crowns and supporting structures, which forms an equilateral triangle with the long axes of the teeth. To produce an image of correct length, the x-ray beam is directed perpendicular to the imaginary line (common side) that bisects the angle formed by the receptor and the teeth. This geometric relationship established with the receptor, structures, and x-ray beam is illustrated in Figure 5–20.

In bisecting angle technique, the receptor is placed closer to the object to be imaged, which permits a reduced source to receptor distance, or use of an 8-inch PID. The angular receptor placements employed with bisecting angle technique require increased vertical angulations when compared with the paralleling technique. Because of the altered vertical angulations, a round PID is recommended for use with bisecting angle technique to minimize

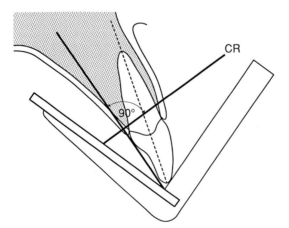

Figure 5–20. Bisecting angle technique requires the receptor to be placed against the lingual surfaces of the tooth crown and supporting structures, which forms an equilateral triangle with the long axis of the tooth. The central ray (CR) is centered and directed at a right angle to the imaginary line that bisects the angle formed by the receptor and the tooth.

cone cut errors. However, the guidelines governing horizontal angulation and centering of the x-ray beam are common to both the paralleling and bisecting angle technique.

The advantage of the bisecting angle technique is that it provides an alternative means of imaging when paralleling technique cannot be used. It is most applicable to situations in which the patient's oral anatomy or behavior prohibits parallel placement of the receptor. Such instances include a shallow palate, a short lingual frenum, the presence of large palatal or mandibular tori, or inability to comprehend the procedure. In addition, the bisecting angle technique can be used to image teeth that are longer than the film by increasing the vertical angulation and, in effect, foreshortening the image enough to record the teeth apices. The disadvantage of the bisecting angle technique is that the recorded image is not as accurate as that produced with the paralleling technique.

Bisecting Angle Instruments

Several bisecting angle receptor holders are available for maintaining the receptor position inside the patient's mouth (Fig. 5–21). The recommended devices are those that provide an extraoral PID alignment guide. However, a simple biteblock is commonly used with this technique (Fig. 5–21). Alignment of the x-ray beam is challenging with the biteblock method, but careful attention to receptor placement, vertical and horizontal angulations, and central ray positioning will yield a useful image.

Patient Positioning

The patient's head position is the same as that described for the paralleling technique. However, the patient's head position has a greater influence on image outcome than with the paralleling technique.

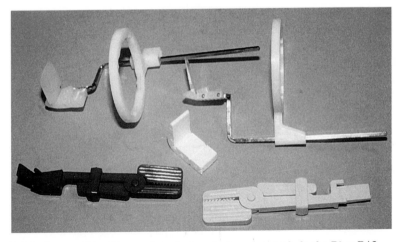

Figure 5–21. Common bisecting angle technique instruments include the Rinn BAI instruments *(top)*; the STABE disposable biteblock *(center)*; and the Snap-A-Ray *(bottom),* all from Rinn Corporation, Elgin, Illinois.

For the maxillary periapical images, the patient's head is positioned so that the midsagittal plane is perpendicular to the floor and the occlusal plane is parallel to the floor. The patient's head is supported by the headrest. For the mandibular periapical images, the headrest is adjusted so that the chin is elevated and the mandibular occlusal plane is parallel to the floor when the patient's mouth is open.

Receptor Placement

The receptor placements are similar to those described for the paralleling technique in terms of the teeth recorded, the horizontal angulations, and centering of the x-ray beam over the receptor. The primary alteration in the bisecting angle technique is in the vertical orientation of the receptor. Rather than placing the receptor parallel to the structures to be imaged, the receptor is placed in an angular position, which forms the equilateral triangle.

Traditionally, a size 2 receptor is used with a 14-periapical image format (6 vertical anterior views and 8 horizontal posterior views) in bisecting angle technique surveys.

Vertical Angulation

Accurate evaluation of the bisecting angle is necessary to determine the correct vertical angulation for each exposure (Table 5–1). Overangulation in the vertical plane will result in foreshortening of the image, whereas underangulation will result in elongation of the image. To reduce vertical angulation errors, the operator can employ starting angulations that are estimates of the bisecting angle for each periapical view.

BITEWING IMAGE PRODUCTION

The bitewing radiographic examination records the maxillary and mandibular crowns of posterior teeth and the alveolar bone crests. A quality bitewing image allows inspection of the interproximal surfaces of the teeth and the alveolar bone crests. Bitewing images are especially useful in the detection of carious lesions on the proximal surfaces of the teeth, secondary caries around existing restorations, and changes in the alveolar crestal bone.

Table 5–1. Bisecting Angles for Periapical Views

Periapical View	Maxilla	Mandible
Incisors	+40° to +50°	−5° to −15°
Canines	+45° to +55°	−5° to −15°
Premolars	+30° to +40°	−10° to −15°
Molars	+20° to +30°	+5° to −5°

Periapical film and direct digital imaging sensors can be used for bitewing imaging by applying a bitewing tab or utilizing a bitewing instrument holder to position the receptor. Some radiographic film packets are manufactured with a bitewing tab attached to the exposure side of the film (see Fig. 5–2).

The typical adult bitewing survey consists of four size 2 vertically or horizontally placed bitewing images: one premolar and one molar projection on each side. Occasionally, an adult film-based bitewing survey may consist of two size 3 bitewing images, one on each side of the mouth. The typical child bitewing survey consists of two horizontally placed bitewings. The receptor size (2, 1, 0) used in the child bitewing survey depends on the child's age and dentition and the size of the oral cavity.

Receptor Placement

The receptor placements described in the following paragraphs are for a four-image horizontal bitewing survey using the Rinn XCP bitewing instrument (Figs. 5–22 and 5–23). The posterior bitewing images include coronal views of the distal of the canine, premolar, and molar teeth. Most typically, a size 2 receptor is placed horizontally, with the exposure side of the receptor facing the operator (film dot convexity surface or level, noncontoured sensor surface). The receptor is centered and placed securely into the bitewing instrument biteblock. Bitewing receptors are placed both vertically and horizontally parallel to the crowns of the teeth.

Premolar Bitewing Placements

To place the receptor, the mouth is entered with the receptor surface parallel to the occlusal surfaces of the maxillary premolar teeth. Then, the inferior aspect of the receptor is gently tipped toward the mandible and placed into the floor of the mouth. The receptor is placed lingual to the mandibular premolar teeth and the bony ridge, and toward the lateral border of the tongue. Next, the biteblock tab is centered over the occlusal surfaces of the second premolar and first molar teeth. The receptor should extend from the mesial of the canine to the distal of the first molar (Fig. 5–22A). The receptor is positioned both vertically and horizontally parallel to the crowns of the premolar teeth (Fig. 5–22B). While the receptor position is stabilized, the patient should be instructed to close slowly but gently onto the bitewing tab surface. If the patient is unable to close onto the tab, the receptor has been placed too close to the teeth. Once the receptor has been placed, the x-ray beam can be aligned with the extraoral PID alignment guide (Fig. 5–22C). The x-ray beam is directed perpendicular to crowns and receptor as well as centered over the receptor site.

Molar Bitewing Placements

To place the receptor, the mouth is entered with the receptor surface parallel to the occlusal surfaces of the maxillary molar teeth. Then, the

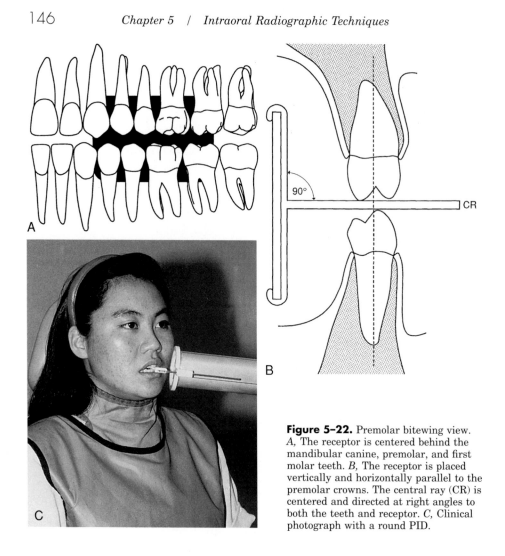

Figure 5-22. Premolar bitewing view. A, The receptor is centered behind the mandibular canine, premolar, and first molar teeth. B, The receptor is placed vertically and horizontally parallel to the premolar crowns. The central ray (CR) is centered and directed at right angles to both the teeth and receptor. C, Clinical photograph with a round PID.

inferior aspect of the receptor is gently tipped toward the mandible and placed into the floor of the mouth. The receptor is placed lingual to the mandibular molar teeth and the bony ridge, and toward the lateral border of the tongue. Next, the bitewing tab is centered over the occlusal surface of the second molar tooth. The receptor should extend from the mesial of the first molar to the distal of the third molar or last erupted molar (Fig. 5-23A). The receptor is positioned both horizontally and vertically parallel to the crowns of the molar teeth (Fig. 5-23B). The remainder of the procedure is similar to that for premolar bitewing placement.

Tab Bitewing Technique

Another approach to bitewing imaging is the tab bitewing technique. The film or sensor may be fitted with a bitewing tab or loop instead of a receptor bitewing device (see Fig. 5-2). Typically, the tab is placed to the center of the receptor to mark the position of the central ray. The receptor is placed lingual

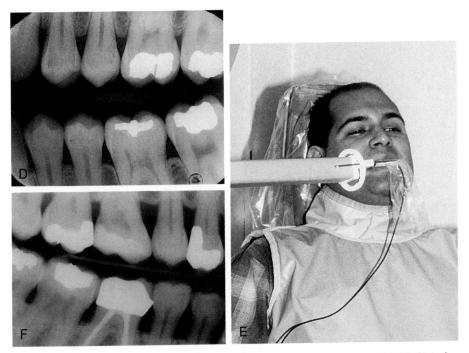

Figure 5–22 *Continued. D,* Bitewing radiograph of the left premolar region. *E,* DDI clinical photograph with a rectangular PID. *F,* DDI bitewing of the right premolar region.

to the mandibular teeth and the bony ridge, and toward the lateral border of the tongue. The tab is centered over the occlusal surfaces of the second premolar and first molar teeth for the premolar projections. For the molar projections, the tab is centered over the occlusal surface of the second molar tooth. The tab is secured with the operator's index finger. The patient is instructed to close slowly but gently onto the bitewing tab surface. As the patient closes, the finger should be rolled into the patient's cheek to avoid injury.

Strict attention to the alignment of the PID is necessary to produce a quality bitewing image. The vertical angulation for the tab bitewing technique ranges from $+5°$ to $+10°$. The horizontal angulation is directed perpendicular to the horizontal plane of the crowns of the teeth in occlusion, and the central ray is directed toward the bitewing tab. To avoid cone cut errors, it is helpful to place two tabs on the receptor, one on the mesial center of the receptor and one on the distal. This provides an anterior alignment guide for the PID. Also, this approach prevents displacement of the receptor and keeps the occlusal plane centered on the image. Finally, to avoid horizontal overlapping, the lateral edges of the tab can be placed parallel to the interproximal surfaces of the teeth. The anterolateral edge of the tab can be used to align the horizontal angulation of the x-ray beam.

OCCLUSAL IMAGE PRODUCTION

As previously described, an occlusal image records a large portion of the maxilla or mandible that is beyond the scope of a single periapical image.

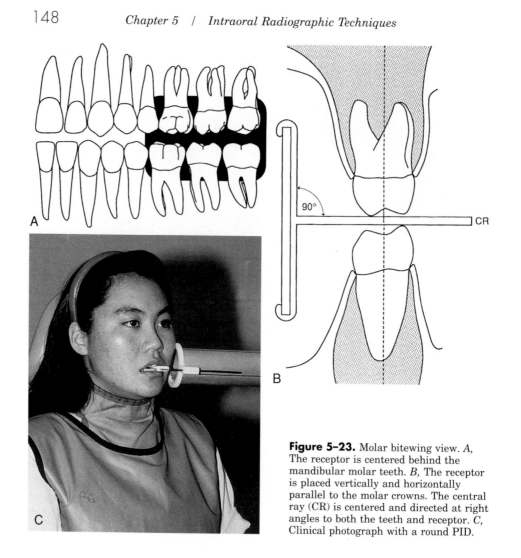

Figure 5–23. Molar bitewing view. *A,* The receptor is centered behind the mandibular molar teeth. *B,* The receptor is placed vertically and horizontally parallel to the molar crowns. The central ray (CR) is centered and directed at right angles to both the teeth and receptor. *C,* Clinical photograph with a round PID.

Usually, occlusal radiographs are taken to supplement other intraoral or extraoral radiographic examinations. The size 4 film receptor (see Figure 5–2) is used for adult occlusal radiography, whereas the size 2 receptor is used for children. Round PIDS are used in occlusal radiography to minimize cone cut errors.

Recall the two types of occlusal projections: topographical and cross-sectional. Topographical projections are frequently used to view a broader area of the maxilla or mandible, impacted teeth, or a large bony lesion, or as a replacement for anterior periapicals in children or adults with restricted opening of the mouth. Topographical occlusal radiography is based on the principles of the bisecting angle technique. Cross-sectional occlusals are most typically used to localize objects such as supernumerary or impacted teeth, foreign objects, or salivary stones in the sublingual and submandibular glands, or to determine mediolateral expansion of the jaws or the displacement of fractures of the maxilla and mandible. Cross-sectional occlusal radiography requires the x-ray beam to be directed perpendicular to the film.

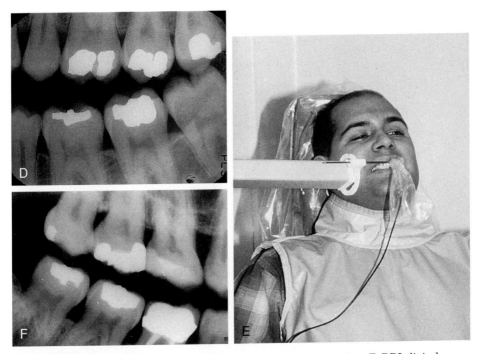

Figure 5-23 *Continued. D,* Bitewing radiograph of the left molar region. *E,* DDI clinical photograph with a rectangular PID. *F,* DDI bitewing of the right molar region.

Maxillary Occlusal Radiography

The receptor is oriented either in the horizontal or vertical plane and placed against the occlusal surfaces of the maxillary teeth. The exposure side of the occlusal film is the plain white side of the packet earmarked by the film identification dot convexity. The dot convexity should be oriented toward the labial aspect of the image. Maxillary occlusal projections are illustrated in Figures 5–24 to 5–26.

Topographical Maxillary Anterior Occlusal

The patient's head is positioned with the midsagittal plane perpendicular to the floor and the occlusal plane parallel to the floor. The dot convexity or white surface of the film is placed against the occlusal surfaces of the maxillary teeth. Approximately 1 cm of the film should extend beyond the labial surfaces of the anterior teeth. The patient gently closes onto the film to maintain its position. A +60° to +65° vertical angulation is used, with the horizontal angle directed perpendicular to the maxillary central incisor teeth and the central ray entering just above the tip of the nose (Fig. 5–24A–C).

This projection shows all the maxillary teeth, but the anterior teeth images are the most comparable to periapical images. In addition, numerous structures are recorded, including the palate, nasal structures, maxillary sinus cavities, zygomatic processes of the maxilla, and nasolacrimal canals (Fig. 5–24D).

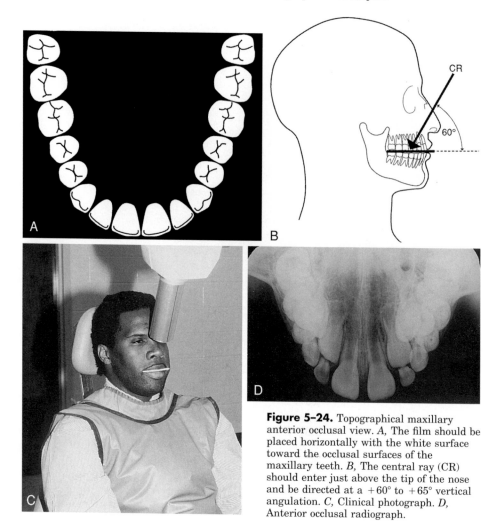

Figure 5–24. Topographical maxillary anterior occlusal view. *A,* The film should be placed horizontally with the white surface toward the occlusal surfaces of the maxillary teeth. *B,* The central ray (CR) should enter just above the tip of the nose and be directed at a +60° to +65° vertical angulation. *C,* Clinical photograph. *D,* Anterior occlusal radiograph.

Topographical Maxillary Posterior Occlusal

The patient's head is positioned with the midsagittal plane perpendicular to the floor and the occlusal plane parallel to the floor. The film is oriented vertically and placed toward the side of interest. The dot convexity or white surface of the film is placed against the occlusal surfaces of the maxillary teeth. Approximately 1 cm of the film should extend beyond the buccal surfaces of the posterior teeth. The film is guided posteriorly until it contacts the ramus. Then, the patient gently closes onto the film to maintain its position. A +60° to +65° vertical angulation is used, with the horizontal angle directed perpendicular to the premolar teeth and the central ray entering 2 cm below the pupil of the eye (Fig. 5–25A–C).

This projection shows one quadrant of the maxillary teeth and alveolar ridge. In addition, numerous structures are recorded, including the nasal fossa, the maxillary sinus, the zygomatic process, and the maxillary tuberosity (Fig. 5–25D).

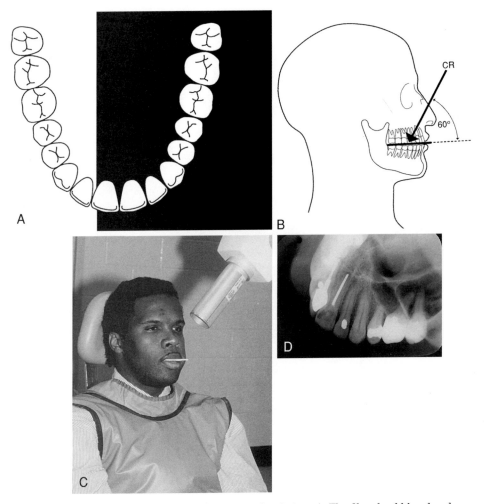

Figure 5–25. Topographical maxillary posterior occlusal view. *A,* The film should be placed vertically with the white surface toward the occlusal surfaces of the maxillary posterior teeth on either the right or left side. *B,* The central ray (CR) should enter 2 cm below the pupil of the eye and be directed at a +60° to +65° vertical angulation. *C,* Clinical photograph. *D,* Posterior occlusal radiograph.

Cross-Sectional Maxillary Occlusal

The patient's head is positioned with the midsagittal plane perpendicular to the floor and the occlusal plane parallel to the floor. The dot convexity or white surface of the film is placed against the occlusal surfaces of the maxillary teeth. Approximately 1 cm of the film should extend beyond the labial surfaces of the anterior teeth. The patient gently closes onto the film to maintain its position. The vertical angulation is determined by directing the beam through the long axes of the anterior teeth. The horizontal angulation is centered with the midsagittal plane, and the central ray enters the skull 1 cm posterior to the bregma, the junction of the sagittal and coronal sutures (Fig. 5–26A–C).

This projection produces a peculiar image, for it depicts all the maxillary

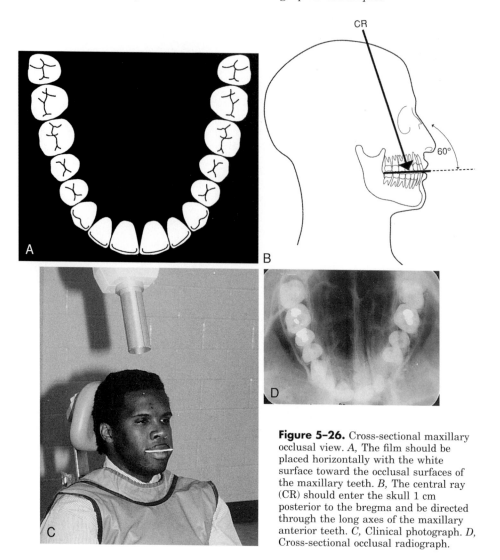

Figure 5–26. Cross-sectional maxillary occlusal view. *A,* The film should be placed horizontally with the white surface toward the occlusal surfaces of the maxillary teeth. *B,* The central ray (CR) should enter the skull 1 cm posterior to the bregma and be directed through the long axes of the maxillary anterior teeth. *C,* Clinical photograph. *D,* Cross-sectional occlusal radiograph.

teeth through the long axes dimension. In addition, some midline structures of the maxilla are imaged. This film is most useful for localizing an impacted or supernumerary tooth (Fig. 5–26*D*).

To penetrate the cranium and produce a maxillary cross-sectional image, the exposure factors should be set at 90 kVp, 15 mA, and a 1.5-second exposure time using E-speed film.

Mandibular Occlusal Radiography

The receptor is oriented either in the horizontal or vertical plane and placed against the occlusal surfaces of the mandibular teeth. The exposure side of the occlusal film is the plain white side of the packet earmarked by the film identification dot convexity. The dot convexity is oriented toward the labial aspect of the image. Mandibular occlusal projections are illustrated in Figures 5–27 to 5–29.

Topographical Mandibular Anterior Occlusal

The patient's head is positioned with the midsagittal plane perpendicular to the floor and the head tilted back so that the occlusal plane is 45° above horizontal (Fig. 5–27A,B). The dot convexity or white surface of the film is placed against the occlusal surfaces of the mandibular teeth. Approximately 1 cm of film should extend beyond the labial surfaces of the anterior teeth. The patient gently closes onto the film to maintain its position. A − 10°

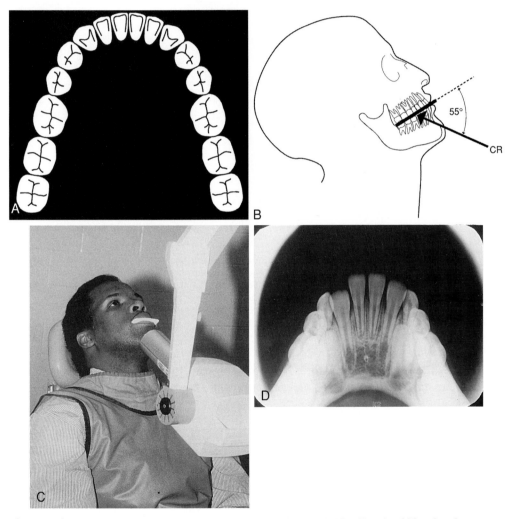

Figure 5–27. Topographical mandibular anterior occlusal view. *A,* The film should be placed horizontally with the white surface toward the occlusal surfaces of the mandibular teeth. *B,* With the occlusal plane 45° above the horizontal, the central ray (CR) should enter through the mentum and be directed at a − 10° vertical angulation. The x-ray beam will have a − 55° angulation to the film. *C,* Clinical photograph. *D,* Anterior occlusal radiograph.

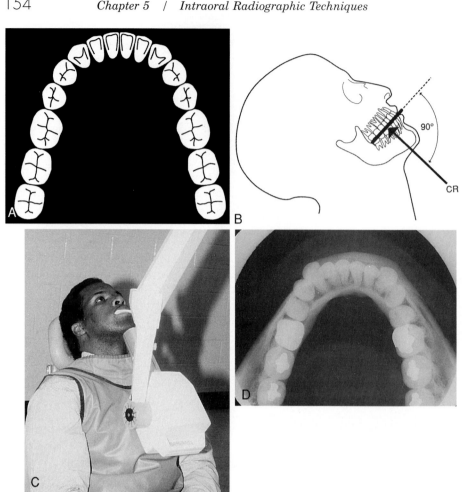

Figure 5–28. Cross-sectional mandibular anterior occlusal view. *A,* The film should be placed horizontally with the white surface toward the occlusal surfaces of the mandibular teeth. *B,* With the occlusal plane nearly 90° above horizontal, the central ray (CR) should enter through the midline of the floor of the mouth and be directed at a −90° vertical angulation. *C,* Clinical photograph. *D,* Cross-sectional occlusal radiograph.

vertical angulation is used, with the horizontal angle directed perpendicular to the mandibular central incisor teeth and the central ray directed through the chin point, or mentum (Fig. 5–27*C*). The x-ray beam will have a −55° angulation to the film (Fig. 5–27*B*).

This projection records the anterior mandible from canine to canine, the mental ridge, and the inferior cortical border of the mandible (Fig. 5–27*D*).

Cross-Sectional Mandibular Anterior Occlusal

The patient's head is positioned with the midsagittal plane perpendicular to the floor and the head tilted back so that the occlusal plane is almost perpendicular to the floor (Fig. 5–28*A,B*). The dot convexity or white surface of the film is placed against the occlusal surfaces of the mandibular teeth. Approximately 1 cm of film should extend beyond the labial surfaces of the anterior teeth. The patient gently closes onto the film to maintain its position. The central ray is directed perpendicular to the film and through the midline of the floor of the mouth (Fig. 5–28C).

This projection records the mandibular teeth through the long axes dimension. In addition, the soft tissue of the floor of the mouth, the buccal and lingual plates of the mandible, the anterior mandible from canine to canine, and the inferior cortical border of the mandible are imaged (Fig. 5–28D). Often, a cross-sectional anterior occlusal is taken to view anteroposterior expansion of the anterior mandible or a salivary stone in the sublingual gland.

Cross-Sectional Mandibular Posterior Occlusal

The patient's head is positioned with the midsagittal plane perpendicular to the floor and the head tilted back so that the occlusal plane is almost perpendicular to the floor (Fig. 5–29A,B). The film is oriented vertically and placed toward the side of interest, as far posterior as possible. The dot convexity or white surface of the film is placed against the occlusal surfaces of the mandibular teeth. Approximately 1 cm of film should extend beyond the buccal surfaces of the posterior teeth. The patient gently closes onto the film to maintain its position. The central ray is directed perpendicular to the film and centered 3 cm posterior to the mentum and 3 cm lateral to the midline (Fig. 5–29C).

This projection records one quadrant of the mandibular teeth through the long axes dimension. In addition, the soft tissue of half the floor of the mouth and the buccal and lingual cortical plates of one side of the mandible are imaged (Fig. 5–29D). Often, a cross-sectional posterior occlusal is taken to view mediolateral expansion of the posterior mandible or a salivary stone in the submandibular gland.

COMMON INTRAORAL TECHNICAL ERRORS AND ARTIFACTS

Numerous technical errors can occur if the clinician does not adhere to the tenets of intraoral radiographic technique. Typical errors include those caused by inadequate preparation of the patient, inaccurate placement of the receptor, improper vertical or horizontal angulation, misalignment of the central ray, and exposure errors.

One of the advantages of direct digital imaging is that the visible image appears on the monitor almost instantaneously after exposure of the sensor. This allows immediate evaluation of the image and correction of errors.

Regardless of the imaging method, the radiographer must be able to recognize errors and correct them. Most of the errors presented apply to both film-based and direct digital radiography. Exceptions are noted in the following text.

Patient Preparation Errors

Frequently, errors occur when the patient is not properly prepared for the radiographic procedure. The clinician should take time to explain the procedure to the patient. The patient should be given adequate instructions to elicit cooperation and should remove any metallic head and neck objects that

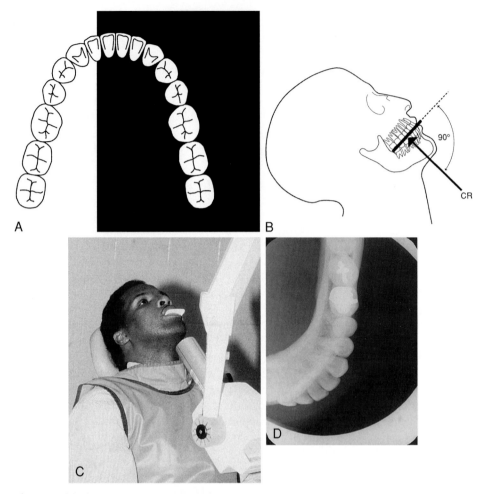

Figure 5–29. Cross-sectional mandibular posterior occlusal view. *A,* The film should be placed vertically with the white surface toward the occlusal surfaces of the mandibular posterior teeth on either the right or left side. *B,* With the occlusal plane nearly 90° above horizontal, the central ray (CR) should enter 3 cm posterior to the mentum and 3 cm lateral to the midline of the floor of the mouth, and be directed at −90° vertical angulation. *C,* Clinical photograph. *D,* Cross-sectional occlusal radiograph.

might interfere with production of a diagnostic image. Movement of the patient or receptor during exposure results in a blurred image (Fig. 5–30). If the movement is minimal, the image may be adequate, but beyond that, the image is best retaken. When prostheses (Fig. 5–31) or eyeglasses (Fig. 5–32) are left in place, these objects superimpose over the teeth and bony structures. In addition, when the thyroid collar is not positioned properly or the head is not positioned to allow the collar to clear the mandible, the thyroid collar will be projected onto the image (Fig. 5–33).

Film Placement Errors

One of most common errors is incorrect receptor placement. Each periapical or bitewing view should contain specific teeth and cover a prescribed region of

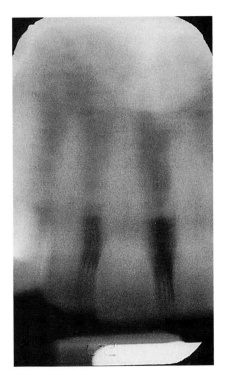

Figure 5–30. Movement of the patient or receptor during exposure produces a blurred image.

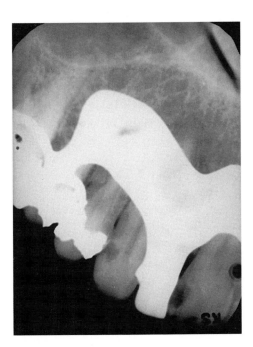

Figure 5–31. A prosthesis was left in place during placement and exposure of this radiograph. The prosthesis is superimposed over the teeth and prevents proper examination of the structures.

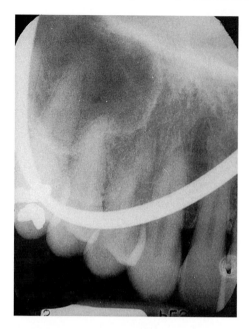

Figure 5–32. The patient should be instructed to remove eyeglasses prior to placement and exposure of the receptor. Otherwise, metallic rim artifacts will be recorded on the maxillary images.

the mouth. Most placement errors occur through inattention to film placement guidelines, which results in inadequate coverage of structures. Another common film placement error results in cutting off the apices of the teeth (Fig. 5–34). This most frequently occurs when the operator places the receptor too close to the teeth or places the biteblock against the opposing teeth, requiring the patient to bite the receptor into place. When the receptor is forced into a position that is too shallow, most of it will extend beyond the crowns of the teeth, which prevents imaging of teeth apices (Fig. 5–34). Another common placement error is backward placement of the receptor. In correct intraoral film packet placement, the film dot convexity and plain white surface of the receptor are positioned toward the x-ray source. When the film packet is reversed, the dot concavity and two-color, lead foil side of the x-ray film are positioned toward the x-ray source. The lead foil partially absorbs the x-ray

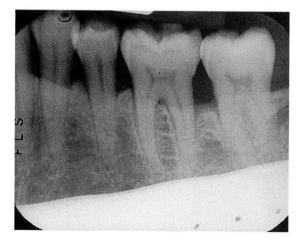

Figure 5–33. The thyroid collar can be projected onto an image if it is not positioned properly or if the patient's head is not positioned to allow the collar to clear the mandible.

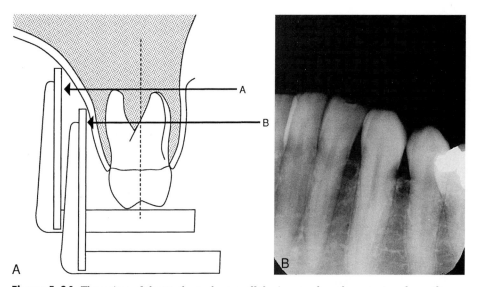

Figure 5–34. The apices of the teeth can be cut off the image when the operator places the receptor too close to the teeth. The diagram shows correct receptor placement *(A)* and incorrect receptor placement *(B)*. The radiograph shows that the apices of the mandibular left lateral canine teeth were cut off because of improper film placement.

beam. As a result, the image orientation is opposite to the side taken, the lead foil pattern is recorded on the film, and a low-density image is produced (Fig. 5–35*A,B*). If the clinician exposes the wrong side of a direct digital imaging sensor, a white or blank image will appear on the video monitor and on the printed image (Fig. 5–35*C*).

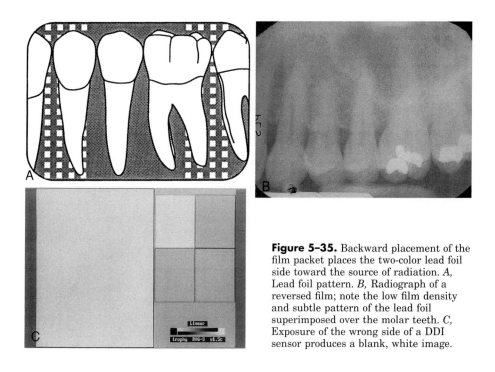

Figure 5–35. Backward placement of the film packet places the two-color lead foil side toward the source of radiation. *A,* Lead foil pattern. *B,* Radiograph of a reversed film; note the low film density and subtle pattern of the lead foil superimposed over the molar teeth. *C,* Exposure of the wrong side of a DDI sensor produces a blank, white image.

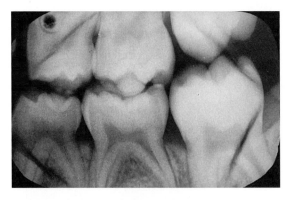

Figure 5–36. Film bending results in black crease artifacts as seen on the corners of this size 0 bitewing film.

Film Handling Errors

The clinician must handle radiographic film so as to avoid film handling artifacts. The most typical artifacts are due to film bending and unintentional film crimping. When the operator bends the edges of films to round the corners for patient comfort, creases are produced in the film emulsion. After film processing, the finished films will display black crease artifacts (Fig. 5–36). Rather than bending film edges, the film should be placed more toward the midline where there is adequate depth, or in some cases, another film size might be more appropriate. The black crescent-shaped artifact shown in Figure 5–37 is produced when the film is crimped or a fingernail indents the film surface during film insertion into a biteblock. The operator should handle the film packet carefully and avoid excessive force when placing the film into a holding device. These artifacts are not produced with direct digital imaging systems owing to the rigid, inflexible nature of the sensor.

Vertical Angulation Errors

The vertical angulation of the x-ray beam controls the long axis dimension of the image. In the paralleling technique, correct vertical angulation positions

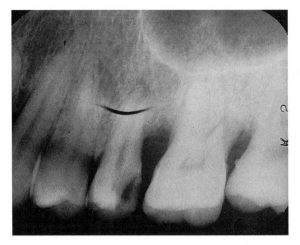

Figure 5–37. A black, crescent-shaped artifact occurs when the film is crimped or a fingernail indents the film surface during insertion of the film into a biteblock.

the x-ray beam perpendicular to the film and to the tooth structure, whereas bisecting angle technique positions the x-ray beam perpendicular to the plane that bisects or divides the angle formed by the tooth and the receptor. In either paralleling or bisecting angle technique, underangulation of the x-ray beam results in elongation or lengthening of the image (Figs. 5–38A and 5–39). To correct errors in image elongation, the operator should increase the vertical angle. Correction of elongation errors of maxillary images requires an increase in the positive vertical angulation, whereas correction of elongation errors of mandibular images requires an increase in the negative vertical angulation (in most clinical situations). Elongation rarely occurs in paralleling technique when paralleling film holding devices are used. However, elongation is not uncommon in bisecting angle technique; it occurs when the clinician aligns the x-ray beam perpendicular to the long axes of the teeth rather than the bisecting angle plane. In addition, an elongated image can be the result of a curved or flexed film edge. The film must be supported lingually by the biteblock so that its surface remains flat during exposure.

In either paralleling or bisecting angle technique, overangulation of the x-

Figure 5–38. The vertical angulation controls the long axis dimension of the image. *A,* Underangulation occurs when the central ray is directed at less than right angles to the tooth and receptor. This results in image elongation. *B,* The correct alignment of the x-ray beam directs the central ray at right angles to both the tooth and receptor. *C,* Overangulation occurs when the central ray is directed at greater than right angles to the tooth and receptor. This results in image foreshortening.

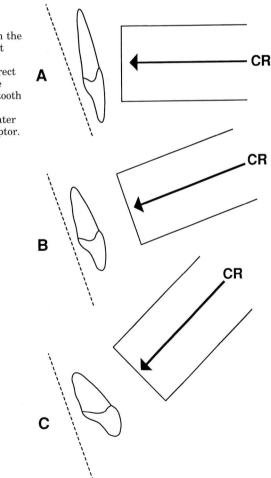

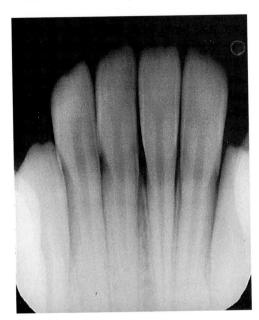

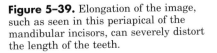
Figure 5–39. Elongation of the image, such as seen in this periapical of the mandibular incisors, can severely distort the length of the teeth.

ray beam results in foreshortening, or a shorter version of the tooth image (Figs. 5–38C and 5–40). To correct errors in image foreshortening, the operator decreases the vertical angle. Correction of foreshortening errors of maxillary images requires a decrease in the positive vertical angulation; correction of foreshortening errors of mandibular images requires a decrease in the negative vertical angulation (in most clinical situations). Foreshortening occurs in paralleling technique when the film is not placed parallel to the long axes of the teeth and results in a bisecting angle type of receptor placement. In bisecting angle, foreshortening occurs when the clinician aligns the x-ray beam perpendicular to the film plane rather than the bisecting angle plane.

Horizontal Angulation Errors

The result of improper horizontal alignment of the x-ray beam is overlapping of the interproximal surfaces of the teeth. This error can occur on either

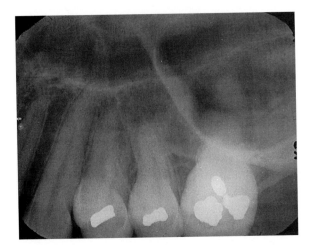

Figure 5–40. Foreshortening of the image results in short, stubby versions of the teeth.

bitewing or periapical images (Fig. 5–41*A,B*). With techniques that utilize holders with extraoral PID alignment guides, this error is due to improper horizontal alignment of the receptor and results in oblique alignment of the horizontal angle of the x-ray beam (Fig. 5–41*C*). In this instance, correction of horizontal overlapping requires the receptor to be placed horizontally parallel to the teeth and thus permits correct horizontal alignment of the x-ray beam (Fig. 5–41*C*). With techniques that do not employ extraoral PID alignment guides, horizontal overlapping is more a function of improper horizontal angulation. The x-ray beam should be directed so that the x-rays will pass through the proximal surfaces of the teeth. If the film is correctly positioned, the x-ray beam should be placed perpendicular to the horizontal plane of the teeth.

Cone Cut Errors

Cone cuts are the result of misalignment of the central ray. When making an exposure, the central ray is positioned over the center of the receptor. When this is not achieved, a portion of the receptor is not exposed. This is

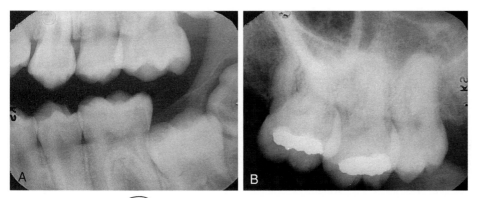

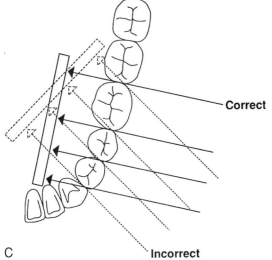

Figure 5–41. Improper horizontal alignment of the receptor or x-ray beam can cause overlapping of the interproximal surfaces of the teeth. This error can occur on *(A)* bitewing or *(B)* periapical images. *C,* With techniques that utilize holders with external PID alignment guides, overlapping is the result of oblique alignment of both the receptor and x-ray beam. Correction of horizontal cylinder overlapping requires the receptor to be placed horizontally parallel to the teeth, which permits correct horizontal alignment of the x-ray beam.

Correct

Incorrect

particularly true with rectangular collimation of the x-ray beam. If the central ray is not both centered and perpendicular to the receptor, cone cuts will be produced (Fig. 5–42). Another possible cause of cone cutting is incorrect assembly of film holding devices with extraoral PID alignment guides. If receptor holders are not properly assembled, the x-ray beam may be incorrectly directed relative to the position of the receptor.

In film-based radiography, a clear zone on the processed film indicates the area of nonexposure (Fig. 5–42C,D). On a direct digital image, the area of nonexposure will appear white. The shape of the cone cut is associated with the type of PID that was used; round PIDs produce curved cuts (Fig. 5–42C), whereas rectangular PIDs produce linear cuts (Fig. 5–42D). To correct a cone cut, the center of the x-ray beam should be moved toward the area of nonexposure in order to recenter the x-ray beam fully over the receptor.

Exposure Errors

Image exposure errors are usually the result of improper exposure settings, inaccurate evaluation of patient stature, or confusion of unexposed films with

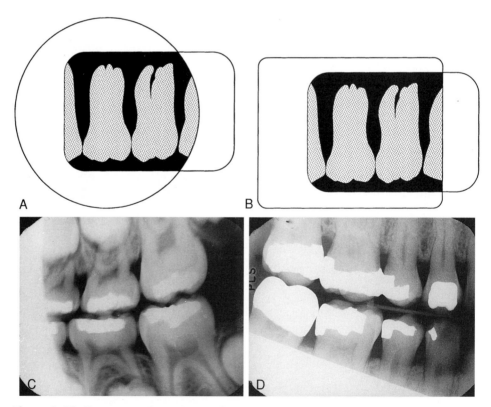

Figure 5–42. Cone cuts or clear zones on the image are the result of misalignment of the central ray. The shape of the cone cut is associated with the type of PID that was used. *A,* A round PID produces a curved cut. *B,* A rectangular PID produces a linear cut. *C,* A bitewing radiograph with an anterior, curved cone cut; *D,* a periapical radiograph with an inferior, linear cut.

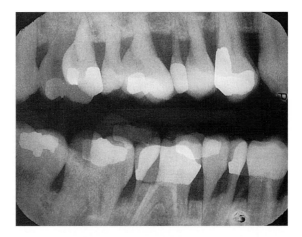

Figure 5–43. A double exposure produces a high-density film with a peculiar pattern due to the superimposition of two images onto one film.

exposed films. The patient's physical size should be evaluated to determine whether any adjustments in exposure time are necessary prior to beginning the imaging procedures. In addition, it is best to set the exposure time prior to receptor placement to ensure that the appropriate exposure time has been selected. With film-based imaging, the operator should employ a systematic method to separate the unexposed film from the exposed film to avoid a double exposure. In Figure 5–43, the film was used twice, with both the premolar and molar bitewing images recorded on one film. The hallmarks of a double exposure are a high-density image, unusual image pattern, and the production of an unexposed film with no image. Correction of a double exposure requires two retakes and special attention given to separation of the unexposed film from the exposed film. A practical separation method places the unexposed film with the white dot convexity surface up and the exposed film with the two-colored dot concavity side up, toward the radiographer. Double exposures cannot be produced with direct digital imaging systems.

In regard to image density, underexposure of the receptor results in a faint, low-density image (Fig. 5–44), whereas overexposure of the receptor results in a dark, high-density image (Fig. 5–45). The image density may be a function of improper exposure factors or lack of consideration of the patient's

Figure 5–44. Underexposure of the receptor results in a faint, low-density image. This example is an underexposed DDI maxillary left molar view.

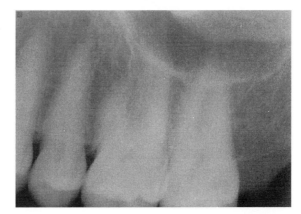

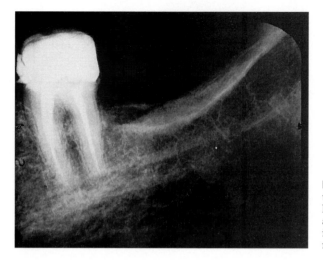

Figure 5-45. Overexposure of the receptor produces a dark, high-density image. This film is an overexposed periapical image of the mandibular left molar region.

physical stature. In addition, low-density images can occur when the operator releases the exposure button prior to completion of the entire exposure cycle.

In direct digital imaging systems that utilize conventional x-ray units, initial exposures are made at the lowest possible timer setting to help the clinician determine suitable exposure factors. Minor aberrations in sensor exposure that result in low- or high-density images can be adjusted during image processing prior to image printing. Frequently, on-screen images differ in density from the actual printed image. A test print will assist the operator in making density adjustments prior to subsequent image printing. However, extreme underexposure or overexposure will result in retakes, just as with film based imaging systems.

DIFFICULT CLINICAL RECEPTOR PLACEMENT SITUATIONS

A number of clinical situations may be encountered that will challenge the radiographer's patient management and technical skills. Anatomical anomalies such as tori, a shallow palate or floor of the mouth, narrow dental arches, and a short lingual frenum may be obstacles to ideal placement of the image receptor. Some patients may experience discomfort in response to receptor placement, whereas others may gag. These reactions to the imaging procedure are disturbing to both the patient and the operator. In addition, radiographic procedures for the edentulous or partially edentulous, disabled, or endodontic patient, or a child, may present unique management and technical problems. Patient management strategies and technique modifications are presented next.

Anatomical Difficulties

Variations in a patient's oral anatomy are not uncommon. However, some anomalies may prevent ideal receptor placement or require selection of an alternative imaging technique. The most common anatomical variations include palatal and mandibular tori, a shallow palate or floor of the mouth, narrow dental arches, and a short lingual frenum.

The torus palatinus, or palatal torus, is a bony protuberance that occurs in the maxillary midline (Fig. 5–46A). The torus mandibularis, or lingual torus, is a bony protuberance on the lingual surface of the mandible near the premolar teeth. Mandibular tori are usually bilateral (Fig. 5–46B). When the tori are small to moderate in size, the paralleling technique can be used. The operator places the apical edge of the receptor lingual to the tori. A size 1 receptor is recommended for imaging the anterior teeth when tori are present. This size will make it easier for the clinician to position and more comfortable for the patient. In addition, the apical edge of the receptor can be covered with a sponge tissue protector to prevent abrasion of the torus (Fig. 5–47). If the tori are large enough to occlude the palate or the floor of the mouth, the bisecting angle periapical technique or topographical occlusal technique may be employed to provide an alternative means of imaging the affected areas of the mouth. In addition, the presence of moderate to large tori may require an increase in the exposure time to produce an image with adequate film density, because of the increased thickness of the bone.

A shallow palate or floor of the mouth may prevent the periapical receptor from being placed parallel to the long axes of the teeth. When this occurs, the paralleling technique can be modified by reducing the vertical angulation of the PID. This will compensate for the lack of receptor parallelism and adjust the angulation to the bisecting plane. This modification is best accomplished

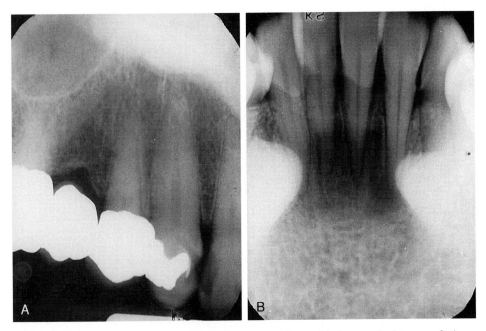

Figure 5–46. Tori have a radiopaque appearance on radiographic images. *A,* A torus palatinus is recorded superior to the apices of lateral incisor, canine, and first premolar teeth on this maxillary right canine periapical. *B,* Bilateral mandibular tori are recorded near the apices of the mandibular lateral incisor teeth on this central incisor periapical.

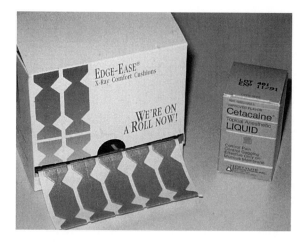

Figure 5–47. The Edge-Ease (Strong Dental Products, Corona, California) tissue protector and topical anesthetic agent such as Cetacaine Topical Anesthetic Liquid (Cetylite Industries, Inc., Long Island City, New York) are useful patient management tools. The Edge-Ease can be placed around the offending edge of the film or sensor. Topical anesthetic agents can be placed on the apical edges of the receptor or onto the tissue protector, or applied to the oral tissues to reduce discomfort or gagging.

with a round PID to avoid cone cut errors. Another option is to use the bisecting angle technique for periapical imaging. A shallow palate or floor of the mouth rarely prevents bitewing imaging of the teeth.

Narrow arches may make anterior periapical placements more difficult. Often the teeth are crowded as well. Usually this problem can be overcome by using the size 1 receptor and placing it as lingual as possible to the teeth to be imaged. If the arch is so narrow that even a size 1 receptor is too wide, topographical occlusal images of the anterior teeth can be produced with either the size 2 receptor or size 4 occlusal film.

A short lingual frenum on the ventral surface of the tongue may prevent the receptor from being seated into the floor of the mouth. In addition, placement against the frenum may be very uncomfortable for the patient. In this situation, the clinician should place a tissue protector onto the receptor to improve apical receptor placement. If that approach is not successful, the receptor should be placed onto the tip of the tongue. When the patient begins to close onto the biteblock, the tongue and the floor of the mouth should relax enough to allow satisfactory receptor placement. This approach may be used for all the mandibular anterior periapicals. The tongue soft tissue will be recorded on the images produced with this technique. Another alternative is to use topographical occlusal radiography to image the area with either the size 2 receptor or the size 4 occlusal film.

Management of Patient Response

The most important aspect of patient management is projection of a confident but empathetic attitude toward the patient and the problem the patient is experiencing. It is best to avoid exaggerated descriptions of receptor placements or references to gagging. Many times the mere suggestion of difficulty increases the patient's anxiety about the imaging procedure. Although one individual may not experience any problems with intraoral imaging procedures, another may find the procedures to be very uncomfortable and difficult to tolerate.

The most common patient complaints involve gagging and pain or discomfort in response to impingement of the receptor edges upon the patient's oral tissues. Receptor placement can be very uncomfortable, especially when the mouth is small or when the palate and floor of the mouth are shallow. This is particularly true of the direct digital imaging sensors that are thicker and more rigid than film. The clinician may find that the patient will be more comfortable if the receptor is placed farther from the tooth structure, where there is more room to allow adequate apical placement of the receptor. Another solution is to place a sponge tissue protector around the offending edge of the film or sensor, as in Figure 5–47. The patient's saliva must be removed from the receptor prior to sponge placement. It is helpful to adapt the tissue protector around the receptor and the apical aspect of the biteblock to eliminate all possible sources of discomfort. In addition, topical anesthetic agents can be placed on the apical edges of the receptor and onto the tissue protector, as well as applied to the oral tissues, to reduce further the discomfort associated with the receptor placement (Fig. 5–47).

Often, the more difficult and challenging management problem is the gagging patient. A small percentage of individuals have an exaggerated gag reflex. Most patients can be helped by use of a preinjection topical anesthetic agent or spray or viscous topical anesthetic agent. Oral anesthetic rinses such as Sensodyne Comfort Rinse (Block Drug Corporation, Jersey City, New Jersey) or Chloraseptic (Richardson-Vicks, Inc., Wilton, Connecticut) can be used to reduce the gag reflex. Other practical desensitizing agents include ice water and salt on the tongue.

Another management measure for the gagging patient is the distraction technique, such as giving the patient a physical task to perform during receptor placement and exposure. The clinician can direct the patient to raise one foot or flex the toes toward the body and maintain either position during the imaging procedure. Often, redirecting or refocusing the patient's attention on the physical task breaks the patient's concentration on the gag reflex. Also, deep breathing through the nose or mouth is helpful to some patients.

If these measures fail, an extraoral radiographic examination may be the only means of gaining the radiographic information needed to evaluate the patient's teeth and supporting structures.

Accommodation of Special Populations

Radiographic procedures for the child, the edentulous or partially edentulous patient, or the disabled patient may present unique management and technical problems. Small oral cavities, primary and mixed dentitions, missing teeth, and inability to cooperate are some of obstacles that might be encountered. Survey, technique, and management suggestions are presented here for imaging these special populations.

RADIOGRAPHIC EXAMINATION OF CHILDREN

Radiographic examination of the child patient may be challenging. Radiographs are often part of the child's first dental appointment. The child may be apprehensive or unable to comprehend the procedure fully. Therefore, it is the responsibility of the clinician to guide the child through the imaging procedure step-by-step and make it as positive an experience as possible.

The selection of appropriate radiographs for the child patient depends on the age, medical and dental history, general oral health, presence of caries, risk factors, and time elapsed since the last radiographic examination. The survey should be based on a thorough clinical examination and the principles of selection criteria. Because children are more sensitive to irradiation, the minimum number of images should be taken to reduce unnecessary exposure. Radiation protection and exposure reduction measures are utilized as with adults. In addition, exposure factors should be appropriate for the child's size and usually require a reduction.

Patient Management

A positive, friendly attitude is a necessary component for managing all patients, especially children. The clinician should speak at eye level and involve the child in conversation. Generally, children respond well to inquiries regarding school activities, hobbies, and pets. Euphemisms or word substitutes can be used to explain procedures to children: x-ray head becomes camera, receptor becomes picture. The operator should take the time to acquaint the child with the new surroundings and explain the procedures in terms and euphemisms appropriate for the child's age. A show and tell approach is a useful method to prepare the child for the task. The clinician should disregard minor inappropriate behavior and reinforce appropriate behavior. In addition, patience and perseverance are required as several step-by-step explanations and placement attempts may be needed before success is achieved. Firm commands and voice control can be used to get the child's attention. A reward for good behavior can be given to the child after completion of the appointment. Various trinkets are available for this purpose. Rewards can produce very positive results and be a pleasant reminder of a job well done.

The clinician should be organized and expedite the procedure by setting the exposure factors and placing the x-ray head in the approximate alignment position before placing the receptor in the mouth. This will help eliminate movement errors. Also, the previously described tissue sponges, topical anesthetics, and distraction techniques will be useful adjuncts for managing the child patient.

Receptor Selection

The size 0 receptor is most frequently used for imaging the primary dentition and mixed dentition to approximately age 7 years. Size 1 or 2 is more appropriate for the child 8 years or older. The size 2 receptor is preferred for child occlusal radiography. The condition of the dentition, size of the oral cavity, and the child's behavior are useful indicators of appropriate receptor selection.

The paralleling technique is preferred for periapical imaging. Trimmed or smaller biteblocks can be used to accommodate the smaller receptor sizes and the size of the child's mouth. Bisecting angle technique and occlusal radiography are useful when paralleling technique cannot be used.

Surveys for the Primary Dentition, Ages 3 to 6 Years. If all surfaces of the teeth can be examined clinically, no radiographs are indicated. If the proximal surfaces of the posterior teeth cannot be inspected clinically, bitewings should be taken. The bitewing survey will consist of two size 0 bitewing images similar to the adult premolar placement. If caries are detected clinically or radiographically, bitewings are repeated at 6-month intervals until no carious lesions are found. If the child has no caries or other risk factors, bitewings can be taken at 12- to 24-month intervals. In addition, anterior occlusals of the erupting permanent teeth and posterior periapicals may be indicated. Usually a maxillary and a mandibular anterior occlusal taken in addition to the bitewings provides an adequate survey (Fig. 5–48A). Size 0 or 1 periapicals can be added when indicated. Another survey option includes bitewings and a panoramic image.

Transitional or Mixed Dentition, Ages 7 to 12 Years. Size 1 or 2 bitewings should be taken at the same intervals as described for the primary dentition. If a more complete radiographic examination is indicated, selected periapicals or a child full mouth survey can be taken. Size 1 or 2 receptors can be utilized to image the dentition. A typical complete or full mouth survey for the child may consist of 12 images: two incisor views, four lateral incisor/canine views, four premolar-molar views, and two bitewings (Fig. 5–48B). Either the paralleling or the bisecting angle technique can be used, whichever is the most appropriate for the clinical situation. Some clinicians substitute an occlusal view for the six anterior views, which results in an eight-image survey: two anterior occlusals, four premolar-molar views, and two bitewings. Another survey option includes bitewings and a panoramic image.

RADIOGRAPHIC EXAMINATION OF EDENTULOUS OR PARTIALLY EDENTULOUS PATIENTS

Patients who are missing some or all of their teeth may present some difficulties for the radiographer. Decreased alveolar bone height and missing or migrated teeth can make receptor placement and retention less than ideal.

Periapical surveys can be taken in either circumstance and usually require fewer images. Typical edentulous or partially edentulous intraoral surveys consist of 10 to 14 periapical views (Fig. 5–49). The survey should include images of the incisor, canine, premolar, and molar regions, including the maxillary tuberosities and the external oblique ridges.

The paralleling technique is the preferred imaging method for evaluation of alveolar bone height and its relationship to the surrounding anatomical structures. To achieve parallel placement of the receptor to the bony ridge, cotton rolls are placed on each side of the biteblock to substitute for missing teeth, resorbed ridges, and lack of opposing teeth. The cotton rolls are secured onto the biteblock with a small or orthodontic rubber band. If the patient has a removable prosthesis, it can be used in opposition to the biteblock and

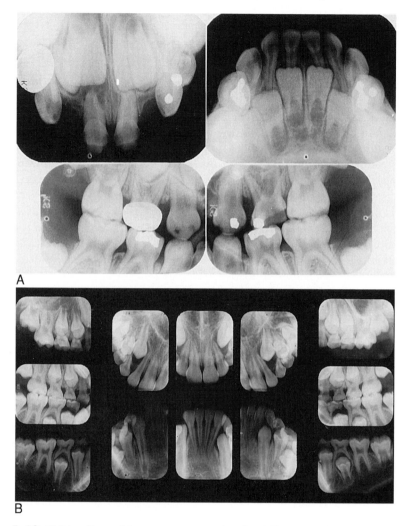

Figure 5–48. Child radiographic surveys may consist of a 4-film survey for the primary dentition *(A)* or a 12-film survey for the mixed dentition *(B)*.

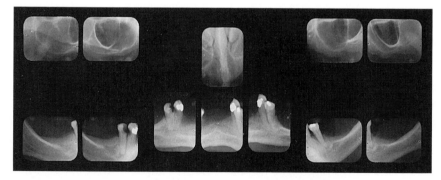

Figure 5–49. Typical intraoral partially or totally edentulous surveys consist of 10 to 14 periapical views. A 12-film, partially edentulous survey is shown here.

assist in receptor placement and retention. However, the prosthesis should be removed for imaging the arch in which it is worn. If the anterior segments of the arches are severely resorbed, topographical occlusals can be substituted for the anterior periapicals. Additional survey options for the partially edentulous patient include selected periapicals of the remaining teeth and a panoramic image. Panoramic radiography is especially useful for imaging the edentulous patient.

DISABLED PATIENTS

Disabled individuals are persons with a mental, physical, medical, or social condition that interferes with normal functioning. In most situations, the clinician will be able to manage the patient and complete the radiographic examination. In treating the disabled person, the radiographer should be patient, understanding, and flexible. In some instances, the patient may require assistance in order to maintain the receptor placement and hold still. An attendant, parent, or staff member may be able to provide this assistance. The helper should be protected by a lead apron, thyroid collar, and gloves, as well as given specific instructions on how to help. If the patient is not able to tolerate intraoral imaging, an extraoral projection may be the best alternative. If not able to cooperate adequately for the extraoral projection, the patient should be referred to a pediatric dentist or a dental professional trained in the management of the disabled.

Endodontic Radiography

Periapical imaging is an integral part of the endodontic treatment of nonvital teeth. Quality images are needed for diagnosis, treatment, and follow-up evaluation. Obstacles to accurate imaging include the presence of the rubber dam, rubber dam clamp, and root canal files. Despite these obstacles, dimensionally accurate images are essential.

The paralleling technique is the method of choice because of its image accuracy. Numerous holding devices are available to maintain parallel placement of the receptor and to enable the clinician to work around the obstacles (Fig. 5–50). Several have extraoral PID alignment guides to direct the x-ray beam. When used correctly, these holders help reduce dimensional and cone cut errors. If parallel placement of the receptor cannot be achieved, the bisecting angle technique can be used. However, the clinician must be aware that the image will be dimensionally distorted.

The size 2 receptor is recommended for endodontic imaging. The receptor is centered over the tooth to be imaged. Sometimes, it is useful to orient the receptor vertically in all regions of the mouth to ensure adequate apical coverage of the tooth. Usually, several images are required during endodontic therapy: preoperative, working, or file length views, and the final fill of the canal(s) (Fig. 5–51). Multirooted teeth may require additional images taken at different horizontal angulations of projection to separate the roots.

Direct digital imaging is very useful in endodontics. Visible images are produced almost immediately on the monitor and provide the information

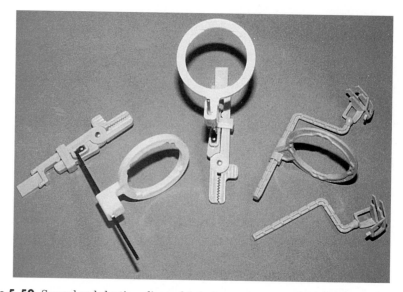

Figure 5–50. Several endodontic radiographic instruments are available for film-based imaging. The Snapex System (Dunvale Corporation, Gilberts, Illinois) *(left)* provides an external PID alignment guide. The EndoRay I and EndoRay II (Dentsply/Rinn, Elgin, Illinois) *(right)* provide either an extension arm or an external PID alignment guide.

necessary to move through the endodontic procedure without film processing interruptions and delays. Figure 5–52 shows a series of such images on tooth number 13. In addition, the patient is anesthetized and better able to comply with the receptor placements.

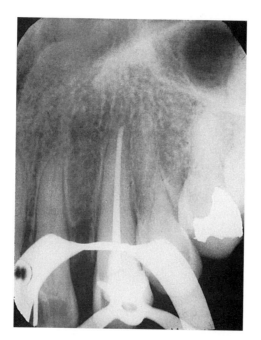

Figure 5–51. The rubber dam and rubber dam clamp are obstacles encountered in endodontic imaging. This maxillary left periapical film records the final fill of the canine root canal.

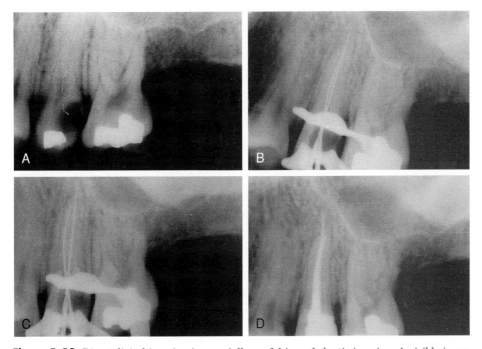

Figure 5–52. Direct digital imaging is especially useful in endodontic imaging. A visible image is produced almost instantaneously on the monitor and provides the information needed to move through the endodontic procedure more efficiently. A typical endodontic image series may consist of a preoperative view *(A)*, a file length view *(B)*, a second file length view at a different horizontal angle to separate the canals of multirooted teeth *(C)*, and a final fill view of the treated root canals *(D)*. (Courtesy of Dr. Cecil E. Brown, Jr., Indiana University School of Dentistry, Indianapolis.)

LOCALIZATION TECHNIQUES

Dental images are two-dimensional representations of three-dimensional objects. Frequently, it is necessary to be able to determine three-dimensional information from radiographs to locate objects such as an impacted tooth or foreign body. There are two basic methods for localizing objects and obtaining the needed three-dimensional information: the tube shift technique and the right angle technique. Both techniques require at least a two-image comparison, with each image taken at a different angle of projection. Many times an existing radiographic survey will provide sufficient information to localize an object.

The tube shift technique compares the change in position of an object between two images taken at different horizontal or vertical angulations. This technique is often referred to as the *Buccal Object Rule,* or *Clark's Rule* (Dr. C. A. Clark described this technique in 1910). The acronym SLOB (S = same; L = lingual; O = opposite; B = buccal) describes the movement of the object from one image to the next relative to the movement of the x-ray head (not the PID). Typically, a change in horizontal angulation (Figs. 5–53 and 5–54) is used with the tube shift method of localization; however, a vertical angulation change will be just as effective (Figs. 5–55 and 5–56).

The first image is taken in a conventional manner, with the x-ray beam

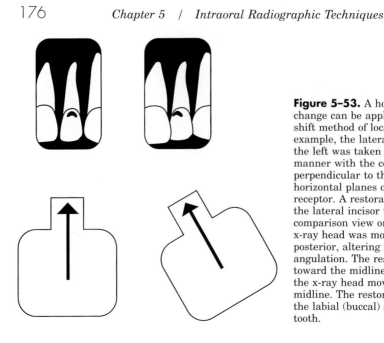

Figure 5-53. A horizontal angulation change can be applied to the tube shift method of localization. In this example, the lateral incisor view on the left was taken in a conventional manner with the central ray directed perpendicular to the vertical and horizontal planes of the teeth and the receptor. A restoration is recorded on the lateral incisor tooth. In the comparison view on the right, the x-ray head was moved toward the posterior, altering the horizontal angulation. The restoration moved toward the midline *(opposite)* while the x-ray head moved away from the midline. The restoration is located on the labial (buccal) surface of the tooth.

placed perpendicular to the receptor and teeth. The second image is taken with at least a 20° angulation change in either the horizontal or vertical plane (Figs. 5–54 and 5–56). If the object moves in the same direction as the x-ray head, it is lingual in location; if the object moves opposite the direction of the x-ray head, it is buccal in location (Figs. 5–53 and 5–55).

A systematic approach to object localization is mentally to retrace the steps involved in the x-ray head alignment during each of the two images. Imagine

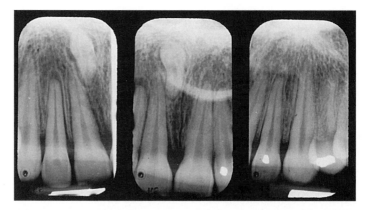

Figure 5-54. In this series of maxillary anterior periapicals, the horizontal angulation changes from film to film. The right lateral incisor view shows a mesiodens (a supernumerary tooth of the maxillary midline) near the apex of the right central incisor. As the x-ray head moves horizontally toward the midline in the central incisor view, the mesiodens moves in the same direction. Thus, the mesiodens is impacted lingually. In addition, the left lateral incisor has a metallic restoration located toward the mesial aspect of the crown. When the x-ray head is moved horizontally away from the midline in the left lateral incisor view, the metallic restoration moves in the same direction. The restoration is located in the lingual pit of the left lateral incisor.

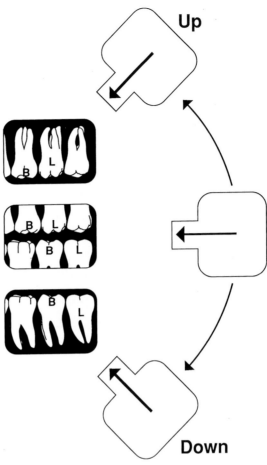

Figure 5–55. A vertical angulation change can be applied to the tube shift method of localization as well. Compare the position of the B (buccal) and L (lingual) letters on the bitewing to the periapical views. When the x-ray head moves either upward toward the maxilla or downward toward the mandible, the letters (objects) change position. Buccal objects move opposite the direction of the x-ray head, whereas lingual objects move in the same direction as the x-ray head.

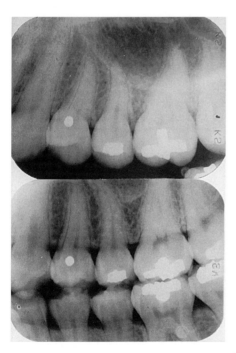

Figure 5–56. In this example of a vertical angulation change, note the position of the metallic restoration on the maxillary first premolar. The restoration moves in the same direction as the x-ray head when the periapical and bitewing films are compared. The restoration is lingual in location. The same process can be applied to the maxillary first molar. The first molar has an occlusolingual (OL) metallic restoration.

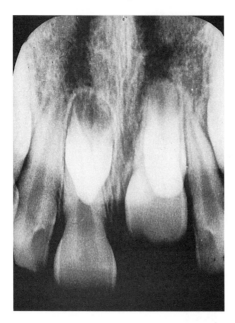

Figure 5–57. The initial film taken in the right angle method of localization is a paralleling technique periapical image. This periapical radiograph shows bilateral mesiodentes (supernumerary teeth of the maxillary midline) superimposed over the maxillary central incisor apices.

the position of the x-ray head relative to the receptor during the first exposure. Then, visualize how the x-ray head was repositioned relative to the receptor during the second exposure. Next, observe the movement of the object in question from the first image to the second image. Sometimes it is useful to compare the location of the object in relation to other structures on the image.

The right angle technique consists of two images taken at right angles to one another. The first image is a conventional paralleling technique periapical projection with the x-ray beam placed perpendicular to the long axes of the teeth (Fig. 5–57); the second image is a cross-sectional occlusal projection

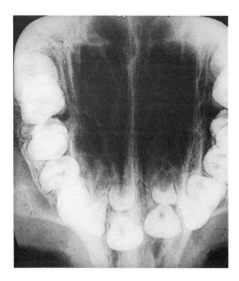

Figure 5–58. The comparison film in the right angle method of localization is a cross-sectional occlusal projection. The maxillary cross-sectional occlusal shows that the mesiodentes are located lingual to the maxillary central incisor teeth.

with the x-ray beam placed perpendicular to the occlusal surfaces of the teeth (Fig. 5–58). Comparison of the two films determines the location of the object(s) in question.

REFERENCES

Ash MM: Wheeler's Dental Anatomy, Physiology and Occlusion, 7th edition, pp 128–307. Philadelphia, WB Saunders, 1993.

Computed Dental Radiography User's Guide. Long Island City, Schick Technologies, Inc., 1994.

Goaz PW, White SC: Oral Radiology: Principles and Interpretation, 3rd edition, pp 151–218. St. Louis, Mosby–Year Book, 1994.

Kasle MJ: Radiography: Cross-fire localization technic. Dent Surv 1969;45:29–31.

Langland OE, Langlais RP, Sippy W, et al: Radiology for Dental Hygienists and Dental Assistants, pp 43–55, 84–126, 159–172. Springfield, Illinois, Charles C Thomas, 1988.

McDonald RE, Avery DR: Dentistry for the Child and Adolescent, 6th edition, pp 32–52, 62–81, 592–615. St. Louis, Mosby–Year Book, 1994.

Miles DA, Van Dis ML, Razmus TF: Basic Principles of Oral and Maxillofacial Radiology, pp 32–52, 73–121. Philadelphia, WB Saunders, 1992.

Owner's Manual and Reference Guide. Sundsvall, Sweden, Regam Medical Systems, 1994.

Successful Intraoral Radiography. Rochester, New York, Eastman Kodak Company, 1990.

Trophy RVG-S User's Manual. Paris, Trophy Radiologie, 1992.

X-rays in Dentistry, pp 40–51, 108–109. Rochester, New York, Eastman Kodak Company, 1985.

6

RADIOGRAPHIC INFECTION CONTROL

GAIL F. WILLIAMSON

Operator Protection

Operatory Preparation

Film Handling Techniques

Processing Procedures

Film Mounting

Cleanup Procedures

Chapter 6 discusses radiographic infection control measures for the operator, radiographic equipment, intraoral image receptors, film processing, film
mounting, and record-keeping procedures. Included in the discussion are
surface disinfection procedures, infection control recommendations for direct
digital imaging and extraoral radiography, and sterilization techniques for
intraoral image receptor instruments. The ultimate goal of the radiographic
infection control protocol is to prevent disease transmission from operator to
patient, patient to operator, and patient to patient.

Dental professionals and dental patients may be exposed to a variety of
microorganisms through direct contact with blood, oral fluids, and secretions,
or indirectly via contact with contaminated surfaces, equipment, and instruments. Intraoral radiographic procedures are not usually associated with the
types of intraoral dental procedures that produce oral fluid aerosols or generate splatters of blood or saliva. Too frequently, radiographic infection control
measures are overlooked, unnecessarily placing both the operator and patient
at risk. During intraoral radiography, the operator's hands and image receptors come in direct contact with oral fluids and microflora, resulting in microbial contamination of the operator and image receptor. Typically, radiographic
procedures are carried out in the same operatories where more invasive

procedures will be conducted, sometimes preceding, during, or following treatments that produce oral fluid aerosols or splatters of blood or saliva.

In addition, improper handling of exposed contaminated film packets can cause further contamination and cross-contamination of darkroom environmental surfaces and processing systems and solutions. Several studies have demonstrated that microbial contamination on radiographic film can survive the processing cycle and that films often become cross-contaminated in the processor. Not only the processed films but also the processing solutions and equipment remained contaminated after processing. Although used developer and fixer solutions will not sustain microbial growth, microorganisms have been shown to survive over a period of 2 weeks. Thus, it is evident that many opportunities for contamination and cross-contamination exist and commonly occur when radiographic infection control measures are breached or inadequately implemented.

Radiographic infection control measures are an integral part of the written dental office exposure control plan and periodic training program as prescribed by the Occupational Safety and Health Administration (Occupational exposure to bloodborne pathogens: final rule, 1991, effective 1992). The following text presents guidelines for radiographic infection control measures that should be practiced and included in the written policy for dental health care professionals.

OPERATOR PROTECTION

Protective clinical attire such as disposable or washable gowns, laboratory coats, clinic jackets, and disposable gloves are mandatory barriers for the operator to prevent contact with oral fluids (Fig. 6–1). Because radiographic procedures do not typically generate aerosols, eyewear and a mask are not generally required. However, protective eyewear with side shields should be worn during manual darkroom processing procedures to avoid chemical injury. Universal precautions (gown, gloves, eyewear, and a mask) are recommended for management of patients with sensitive gag reflexes.

To prepare the operatory, the clinician should wear a gown, eyewear, a mask, and heavy utility gloves during precleaning and disinfection procedures to reduce direct contamination of the skin, mucous membranes, and eyes (Fig. 6–2). The hands should be thoroughly washed with an antimicrobial handwash solution, rinsed, and dried before gloves are donned. Disposable latex or vinyl examination gloves should be worn during all patient care activities that result in direct contact with oral fluids. In addition, the hands should be washed before and after each patient, before glove placement, after glove removal, and after barehanded touching of objects or surfaces likely to be contaminated.

OPERATORY PREPARATION

Surfaces that may be contaminated with saliva during patient radiographic procedures must be precleaned, disinfected, and preferably covered prior to seating the patient. Precleaning procedures are best completed at the begin-

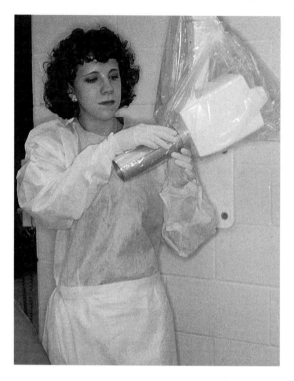

Figure 6–1. During radiographic procedures, the operator should wear protective clinical attire such as the disposable gown seen here, as well as disposable gloves.

Figure 6–2. The operator should wear a gown, eyewear, a mask, and heavy utility gloves during precleaning and disinfection procedures.

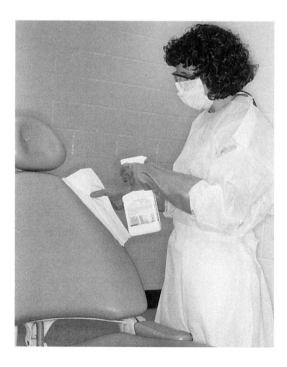

ning of the day using appropriate operator barriers. Environmental Protection Agency–registered and American Dental Association–accepted water-based surface disinfectant-detergents such as chlorine compounds, iodophors, and combination synthetic phenolics should be used to preclean surfaces as well as to provide surface disinfection. The operator should spray the antimicrobial agent thoroughly onto all accessible surfaces or apply it with a wetted paper towel. Then the sprayed surfaces should be vigorously wiped with a fresh paper towel. The precleaned surfaces should be sprayed with the disinfectant again, allowing the solution to remain in contact with the surface for 10 minutes or as prescribed by the manufacturer. Once the surfaces have been precleaned and disinfected, surface covers can be placed for each patient, thus reducing the need for repeated surface preparation throughout the day. However, if the surface becomes contaminated during cover removal procedures, precleaning and disinfection must be repeated prior to placement of fresh surface covers. It is advisable to preclean and disinfect accessible surfaces between patients if the status or preparation of the unit is unknown to the operator.

Unit Protocol

All exposed working surfaces should be precleaned and disinfected as previously described. These surfaces include (1) sink fixtures and countertops; (2) lead shields—apron and thyroid collar; (3) x-ray equipment components: x-ray head, position indicating device (PID), yoke, arms, control panel, exposure button; and (4) chair components: headrest, adjustment controls, arms, back, and seat. Employ the wetted paper towel rather than the spray technique for preparing the x-ray control panel electrical switches, dials, and meters and the chair adjustment control switches.

Clear plastic bags, sheet film or wrap, and tubing are effective surface covers for operatory and x-ray equipment. Appropriately sized plastic bags can be used to cover the x-ray tube head and PID, chair (Fig. 6–3), and lead apron and thyroid collar. Plastic wrap or plastic sheet film is a useful covering

Figure 6–3. Plastic bags are effective surface barriers for the x-ray head and dental chair.

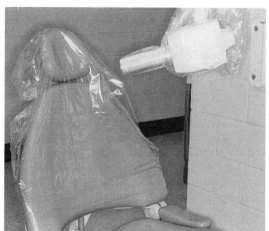

material for countertops and the x-ray control panel, whereas a plastic baggie is an effective cover for the sink fixtures and the exposure button (Fig. 6–4). If such barrier techniques are not employed, precleaning and disinfection procedures must be completed between patients.

Direct Digital Imaging

Direct digital imaging presents the operator with new infection control challenges. With this filmless technology, the image receptor is an intraoral x-ray sensor rather than x-ray film. The sensor is used repeatedly to acquire successive images, and it is connected to the computer hardware processing system via a nonremovable electrical cable. The intraoral sensor and cable cannot be heat sterilized, but some of the sensors can be immersed in a cold sterilant, such as a 2.0% to 3.2% concentration of glutaraldehyde for 10 hours. Because of the prolonged sterilization time, it is recommended that the sensor be covered with plastic tubing prior to intraoral use (Fig. 6–5). The plastic tubing should extend from the sensor to include an adequate length of the cable to avoid direct oral fluid contamination. Care must be taken to maintain the integrity of the plastic tubing around the sensor. Some of the sensor holding devices allow the operator to cover both the sensor and instrument with the plastic tubing. This method depends on the type of sensor holder instrument employed during the imaging procedure. A prepared, covered surface must be available to place the sensor on between exposures.

With direct digital imaging, the operator must be careful to apply the same

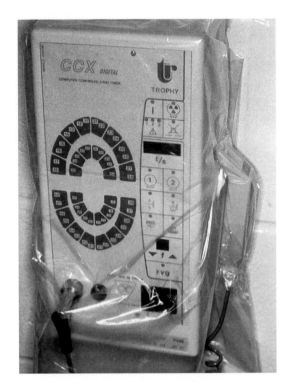

Figure 6–4. The control panel should be covered with plastic wrap or plastic sheet film to allow manipulation of the exposure factors during image acquisition. A small plastic baggie or plastic wrap should be used to protect the exposure switch.

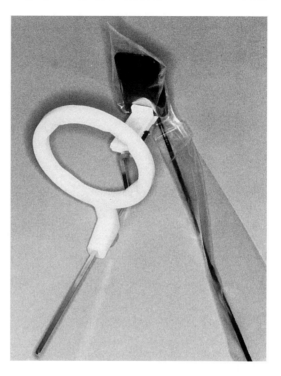

Figure 6–5. Plastic tubing is an effective barrier material for covering the x-ray sensor and cable used in direct digital imaging systems.

types of precautions to preclean, disinfect, and protect the equipment utilized in image acquisition, image processing, and image printing as with conventional radiographic techniques. Some direct digital imaging systems require the use of the conventional x-ray head for sensor exposure and, therefore, necessitate preparation of the dental operatory and radiographic equipment as well as the system hardware (Fig. 6–6). One system is self-contained and includes the x-ray equipment. The covered equipment can be brought into the prepared operatory to acquire, process, and print the digital image (Fig. 6–7).

Extraoral Radiography

Panoramic and cephalometric radiographs are the most typical extraoral radiographs taken in the dental office. Although surface contact with patient saliva is minimal during extraoral radiography, the operator should take appropriate measures to prepare these units for patient procedures. For panoramic units, the operator should preclean, disinfect, and cover the x-ray control panel, exposure button, chinrest, biteblock holder, head positioning guides, and handgrips (Fig. 6–8). Sterilized or disposable biteblocks are preferred for panoramic radiography. Another option is to cover the bitepiece with a plastic barrier. Clean hands should be used to load the cassette in the darkroom and position the cassette on the machine. The hands should be washed and gloved to prepare and position the patient for the procedure. Once the film has been exposed and the patient released, the gloves should be removed and the hands washed prior to handling the cassette for film

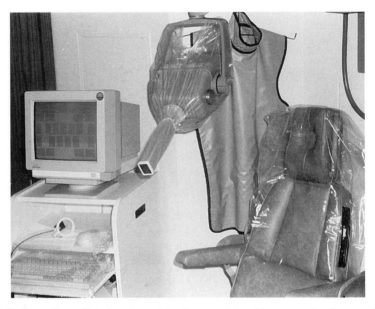

Figure 6–6. Some direct digital systems, like the one pictured here, require the use of conventional x-ray equipment. The operatory and x-ray equipment should be prepared and covered with appropriate surface barriers. In addition, the direct digital imaging system components, such as the x-ray sensor, mouse, keyboard, and counter surface, should be covered in such a way as to prevent saliva contamination during image acquisition.

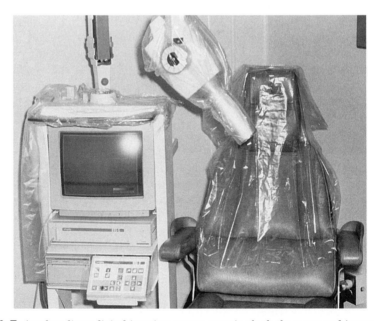

Figure 6–7. Another direct digital imaging system contains both the x-ray and image processing equipment. The x-ray head, exposure control panel, image processing keyboard, sensor, and exposure switch should be precleaned, disinfected, and covered. The top counter of the monitor should be covered to provide a resting place for the sensor and its holder between exposures. The dental chair should be prepared and covered as previously described.

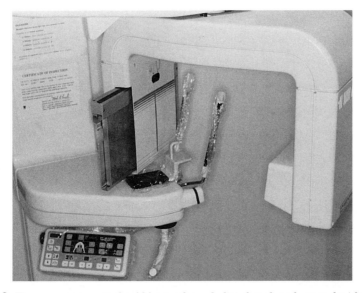

Figure 6–8. The panoramic unit should be precleaned, disinfected, and covered with plastic surface barriers. Components that should be protected include the head positioning guides, chinrest, control panel, and handgrips. A sterilized or disposable bitepiece should be positioned into the chinrest platform.

processing. The preparatory procedures for cephalometric radiography are similar to those previously described. The operator should preclean and disinfect the x-ray control panel, exposure button, cephalostat ear rods, and brackets, as well as the nasion support and orbitale pointer. As a precaution, the exposure panel, exposure switch, and ear rods can be covered with plastic wrap. Cassette loading and handling procedures are the same as described for panoramic radiography.

Radiographic Supplies

All materials necessary for completion of the radiographic procedure should be assembled prior to the seating of the patient. These materials should be either sterilized or disposable. Packaged sterilized receptor holders, cotton rolls, bitewing tabs, prostheses containers, film, a film receptacle, and the like are obtained and placed on a covered surface prior to beginning the procedure (Fig. 6–9). Film supplies can be dispensed in typical survey quantities (20-film full mouth survey or 4-film bitewing survey), along with cotton rolls or bitewings tabs as needed, and placed in a disposable plastic cup or plastic bag. All supplies should be kept in a central supply area and brought to the operatory for use prior to the procedure. The chances for cross-contamination increase when additional materials must be obtained during the appointment. If the necessity arises, contaminated gloves must be removed and the hands washed prior to acquiring the needed materials. Another option for the operator is to enlist the help of another staff member to retrieve the needed items.

Once the operatory has been prepared, the patient can be seated. The

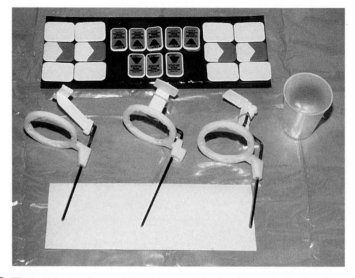

Figure 6–9. The counter surface outside the operatory should be prepared and covered for use during the radiographic procedures. A film mount can be placed under a plastic surface barrier to help organize the survey for the operator. Unexposed films should be positioned with the white side up and exposed films with the colored side up.

medical history should be taken or reviewed prior to exposing an authorized radiographic survey. Because many potentially infectious patients cannot be identified through the medical history or oral examination, it is necessary to treat all patients as potentially infectious and consistently apply the office infection control policy. Then the appropriate entries in the patient record can be made and the record stored away from the treatment area. Another option is to place the record into a plastic cover or envelope to avoid contamination during treatment. The operator avoids handling the patient record with contaminated gloves.

To begin the radiographic procedures, the operator should wash the hands and don disposable gloves, preferably within sight of the patient. All objects and surfaces that will be touched during the procedure should have been sterilized or disinfected by this point. The film or sensor holder instruments are assembled next and the lead apron and thyroid collar placed on the patient.

FILM HANDLING TECHNIQUES

The operator can utilize a variety of film handling techniques to prepare the film packets for exposure and darkroom processing or daylight loader automatic film processing.

With the operator wearing clean gloves, the unexposed films should be arranged in survey format on a covered surface outside the operatory and behind an adequate radiation barrier. To differentiate unexposed and exposed films, the unexposed films should be placed with the white side up and exposed films with the colored side up (Fig. 6–9). The film can also be arranged on top of a film mount placed underneath the plastic surface cover (Fig. 6–9). The saliva should be removed from the film packet with a paper towel after each film exposure is completed. Once all exposures have been made, the films can be placed in a disposable plastic cup or bag or on a clean paper towel for transport to the darkroom. Neither unexposed nor exposed radiographic film should be placed in the operator's gown or laboratory coat pocket because of the potential for contamination and cross-contamination throughout the day.

Another film handling approach employs the use of a barrier device for the film packet. Several manufacturers market a clear plastic envelope with an adhesive seal into which the film can be placed prior to insertion into the patient's mouth (Fig. 6–10A). These barriers are designed to keep the film

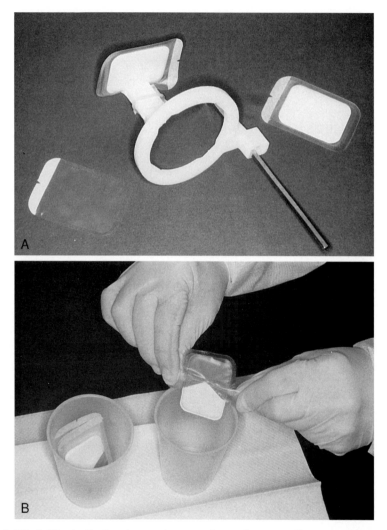

Figure 6–10. *A,* Plastic film barrier envelopes can be used to cover films to prevent saliva contamination during placement and exposure procedures. *B,* With gloved hands, the operator should open the barrier envelope at the tear strip and allow the film packet to drop into a clean receptacle in preparation for film processing.

from being contaminated with oral fluids during placement and exposure procedures. Film barrier covers are recommended for paper-wrapped film packets and daylight loader automatic processing systems. After the covered films have been exposed, the gloved operator should open the plastic pouch at the tear slit and allow the film packet to drop into a clean disposable container or onto a fresh paper towel (Fig. 6–10B). The soiled gloves are removed and the hands washed before proceeding to the darkroom or daylight loader processor.

The film immersion technique is another film handling method that can be used to disinfect radiographic film packets prior to processing procedures. Plastic-covered film packets only (paper-covered film packets will absorb the chemical solution) can be immersed in a 0.5% sodium hypochlorite (bleach) or iodophor solution for 10 minutes. Wearing fresh gloves, the operator rinses the disinfected film packets with water, dries them with a clean paper towel, and places them into a disposable plastic cup or bag for transport to the darkroom or daylight loader automatic processor.

PROCESSING PROCEDURES

After completing the radiographs, the contaminated gloves are removed and the hands washed and covered with a fresh pair of gloves prior to entering the darkroom. Care must be taken to avoid contact with extraneous surfaces such as walls, doors, doorknobs, or other workstations that may be contaminated. A paper towel or a plastic overglove is recommended for entry into the darkroom. The darkroom work surfaces are prepared and covered in the same manner as the operatory surfaces. Waste disposal containers are conveniently located to receive film wrappings, gloves, and used paper towels. Several fresh paper towels are placed on the covered darkroom work surface. For saliva-contaminated films, the cup, bag, or towel containing the exposed films is placed on one of the towels. One film at a time, the operator removes the external plastic wrapping and lead foil and discards them into the disposal container or onto the same paper towel. Then the operator opens the inner black paper wrapping and allows the film to drop out onto the other paper towel, avoiding any contact with the film itself (Fig. 6–11). Once all the films have been dropped out of the packets, the film receptacle and paper toweling with the film wrappings are discarded before the operator removes the contaminated gloves and washes and dries the hands.

With clean hands, the films are handled on the edges and either attached to a manual processing rack (Fig. 6–12A) or inserted into the automatic processor (Fig. 6–12B). If a sink is not available in the darkroom, the operator uses powderless examination gloves to eliminate powder contamination of the film emulsion. In addition, use of double film packets requires the operator to separate the dropped-out films before placing individual films onto a processing hanger or inserting them into the automatic processor. The use of the film drop-out technique keeps the film processing systems free from contamination and from becoming a potential source of cross-contamination. Film packets prepared by the barrier envelope or film immersion technique can be handled without gloves, but it is recommended that the operator

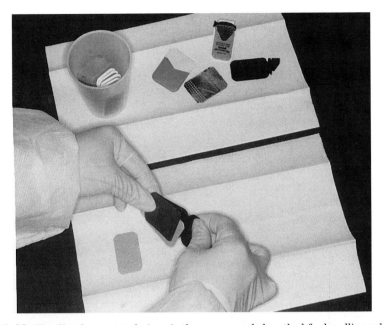

Figure 6–11. The film drop-out technique is the recommended method for handling saliva-contaminated films in the darkroom. The operator should shell the plastic outer wrapping and lead foil onto a separate paper towel or into a disposal container. Then the operator should open the inner black paper wrapping and let the film drop out onto another paper towel without touching the film itself.

wear inexpensive powderless plastic or vinyl gloves as a precaution during processing procedures.

Automatic Processors with Daylight Loaders

Daylight loader processors require a different method of film handling because of their design. These devices are equipped with cloth portals or rubber sleeves that permit insertion of the hands and arms into the unit, as well as a white light window filter and viewing device (Fig. 6–13). The internal working area and window of most units can be disinfected, but because of the restricted internal operational space and the inability to disinfect the insertion sleeves adequately, only uncontaminated films should be processed in these units. The film barrier and film immersion techniques recommended for daylight loader processors have been discussed.

Once the films have been dropped out of the barrier or disinfected, the films are placed into a disposable cup or plastic bag or onto a fresh paper towel. With the operator's clean hands, the daylight loader window is opened, and paper toweling or plastic wrap is placed over the bottom surface of the unit. Next, the film receptacle and powderless examination gloves are placed onto the covered internal surface (Fig. 6–14). Then the lid is closed and the hands inserted through the sleeve portals. Once the hands are inside the unit, the gloves are donned and the films are shelled, handled on the edges, and inserted into the processor. When all films have been inserted, the gloves are

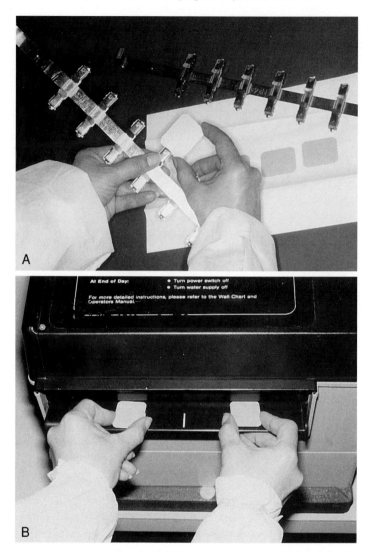

Figure 6–12. The operator should remove the gloves and wash the hands after all films have been dropped out and the wrappings properly discarded. *A,* For manual processing systems, individual films should be attached to a manual processing rack, as shown here. *B,* For automatic processing systems, the films should be inserted into the feed mechanism of the processor. Note that with both techniques the operator handles the films on the edges rather than on the film surfaces.

removed and the hands withdrawn through the sleeves. Finally, the daylight loader window is opened, and the waste materials are enfolded in the bottom covering material and discarded.

FILM MOUNTING

Gloves are shed and the hands washed prior to removing films from the processor or arranging or mounting dental radiographs. The processed films

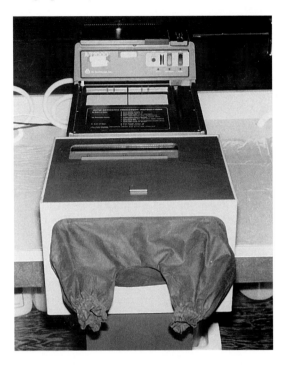

Figure 6–13. A daylight loader automatic processing system with rubber sleeves and a white light filter and viewing window is shown here.

can be organized and arranged on a clean viewbox surface. The films are mounted in a plastic pocket mount that provides protection for the finished radiographs and permits careful disinfection when needed. The mounted survey is displayed on a precleaned and disinfected operatory viewbox. If

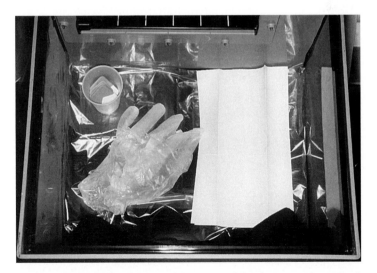

Figure 6–14. The daylight loader box should be prepared for the processing procedures by covering the bottom surface with plastic wrap or paper toweling. The film receptacle and gloves should be placed onto the covered surface through the lid prior to inserting the hands through the access sleeves.

the mounted radiographs are to be referenced during an aerosol-producing procedure, the survey can be further protected by covering the viewbox surface with clear plastic wrap or a plastic bag (Fig. 6–15). In addition, the operator should refrain from handling mounted radiographs with contaminated gloves. These precautions will reduce survey and patient record contamination.

CLEANUP PROCEDURES

The radiographic infection control protocol must allow for the retaking of undiagnostic images. It may be desirable to leave the unit surface covers and instruments intact until the processed films have been examined, especially if difficulties were encountered. Otherwise, the operator will have to re-cover exposed surfaces and assemble new materials to complete the re-exposures.

When the radiographic procedures are finished, fresh gloves are donned to clean up the operatory. Intraoral film and sensor holders are placed in a presoak solution or ultrasonic bath in preparation for instrument sterilization. Disposable materials such as paper towels and cotton rolls are discarded in a plastic-lined waste container. All surface covers are removed without contacting the underlying surface, and these materials are deposited in an appropriate waste container. A convenient cleanup method is to invert the chair bag and insert all other contaminated materials inside it, tie it up, and discard it as previously described (Fig. 6–16). Any surfaces contaminated during treatment, removal procedures, or not protected with surface covers are cleaned and disinfected. However, disinfection of all working surfaces is optimal.

In most locations, the waste generated from radiographic infection control procedures is not considered to be infectious or regulated medical waste. The discarded gloves, surface covers, film wrappings, and paper toweling should be handled with gloves and placed in impervious plastic bags according to local and state regulations. Such discarded items do not require neutraliza-

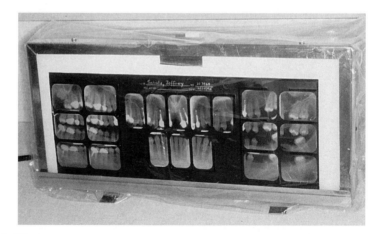

Figure 6–15. The processed survey should be placed in a pocket film mount and positioned under a covered viewbox for reference during an aerosol-producing procedure.

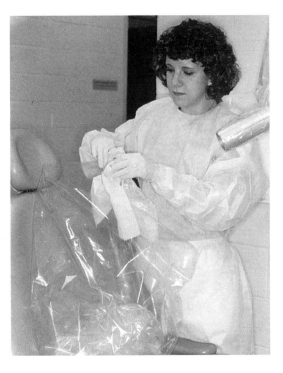

Figure 6–16. A convenient method for unit cleanup is to invert the chair bag and insert all disposable, contaminated materials inside it. Afterward, the bag can be tied up and discarded in an appropriate manner.

tion or special handling. However, it is imperative that every dental office and clinic be familiar and in compliance with current disposal regulations in their area.

Instrument Processing

Instrument processing involves several steps: presoaking, precleaning, and sterilization. The operator should wear protective clothing, eyewear, a mask, and utility gloves during these procedures. Most film and sensor holder instruments can be steam autoclaved. For other heat sterilization methods, the manufacturer's guidelines should be consulted.

Instruments that cannot be cleaned immediately are placed into a holding solution to prevent drying of the saliva. This holding medium can be a germicide or the ultrasonic cleaning solution. Ultrasonic cleaning is preferable to instrument scrubbing for precleaning contaminated holders. The instruments are processed from 4 to 15 minutes in the ultrasonic cleaning solution. Then, the basket of instruments is removed from the solution, rinsed thoroughly with water, and generally dried. The instrument parts are organized into functional groups and sealed in plastic or paper-plastic sterilization bags. The manufacturer's instructions are followed in regard to steam sterilizer loading, time, and temperature requirements. The sterilization cycle is started only after the unit has reached the appropriate temperature.

Some plastic materials used for holder instruments and panoramic biteblocks cannot withstand heat sterilization. However, these materials can be submerged in a 2% to 3.2% glutaraldehyde solution for 10 hours to achieve sterilization. All such items should be precleaned, rinsed, and dried prior to solution submersion. After adequate sterilant exposure, the instruments should be thoroughly rinsed in water and dried. All processed items are handled using aseptic techniques and placed into clean packages for storage.

REFERENCES

American Academy of Oral and Maxillofacial Radiology: Infection control guidelines for dental radiographic procedures. Oral Surg Oral Med Oral Pathol 1992;73:248–249.

American Dental Association; Council on Dental Materials, Instruments, and Equipment; Council on Dental Therapeutics; Council on Dental Research; and Council on Dental Practice: Infection control recommendations for the dental office and the dental laboratory. J Am Dent Assoc 1992; Supplement:1–8.

Bachman DE, White JM, Goodis HE, et al: Bacterial adherence and contamination during radiographic processing. Oral Surg Oral Med Oral Pathol 1990;70:669–673.

Centers for Disease Control: Recommended infection-control practices for dentistry, 1993. MMWR Morb Mortal Wkly Rep 1993;42:1–12.

Cottone JA, Molinari JA: State-of-the-art infection control in dentistry. J Am Dent Assoc 1991;123:33–41.

Glass BJ: Infection control in dental radiology; current and future. NY State Dent J 1994;60:42–45.

Goaz PW, White SC: Oral Radiology: Principles and Interpretation, 3rd edition, pp 219–226. St. Louis; Mosby–Year Book, 1994.

Katz JO, Cottone JA, Hardman PK, et al: Infection control protocol for dental radiology. Gen Dent 1990;38:261–264.

Katz JO, Geist JR, Molinari JA, et al: Potential for bacterial and mycotic growth in developer and fixer solutions (abstract). Dentomaxillofac Radiol 1988; Supplement 10:52.

Miller CH, Palenik CJ: Infection Control and Management of Hazardous Materials for the Dental Team, pp 116–131, 132–147, 168–169, 172–186, 204–209. St. Louis, Mosby–Year Book, 1994.

Neaverth EJ, Pantera EA: Chairside disinfection of radiographs. Oral Surg Oral Med Oral Pathol 1991;71:116–119.

Stanczyk DA, Paunovich ED, Broome JC, et al: Microbiologic contamination during dental radiographic film processing. Oral Surg Oral Med Oral Pathol 1993;76:112–119.

7

DARKROOM FILM PROCESSING AND QUALITY ASSURANCE PROCEDURES

GAIL F. WILLIAMSON

Darkroom Requirements

Processing Systems

Image Transformation

Film Mounting

Film Duplication

Quality Assurance

Film Handling and Processing Artifacts

Darkroom processing and quality assurance procedures apply to film-based imaging. Despite exacting technical and exposure techniques, radiographic images can be rendered inferior or undiagnostic if the processing of the exposed film is not carried out appropriately. Film processing is the second step in image production, carried out after initial x-ray exposure of the film emulsion, which forms the latent image. Film processing changes the latent image into a visible image through chemical interaction with the exposed film emulsion.

Film processing, whether automatic or manual, involves developing, rinsing, fixing, washing, and drying of the film. Usually, these procedures are completed in a darkroom unless the exposed films are processed with a daylight loader automatic processing system.

To produce high-quality finished radiographs, the clinician should be familiar with the processing equipment, chemicals, processing sequence, and maintenance procedures. Those topics are presented here, as well as film mounting, film duplication, and quality assurance procedures. Finally, common darkroom processing errors and their correction are presented as a means of trouble-shooting problems when they occur.

DARKROOM REQUIREMENTS

The darkroom should be designed so that film processing can be carried out in an efficient and precise manner. It should be of adequate size and properly ventilated to provide a reasonable working environment. Darkroom cleanliness is essential to quality processing, for chemical spills and other debris can produce artifacts that degrade the image. Because the processing procedures are completed in almost total darkness, attention should be given to the room design and the placement of the darkroom equipment.

Radiographic film is sensitive to light, temperature, and humidity. It is essential that all white light be eliminated. Common sources of white light leaks include the doorframe, ceiling tiles, vents, and wall seams. Leaks can be sealed with black masking tape or weatherstripping. The relative darkroom temperature should be 70°F (21°C) and the humidity from 50% to 70%. Extreme darkroom temperatures can have a deleterious effect on the processing solutions and their subsequent action on the film emulsion. Low-humidity conditions can cause static electricity problems, whereas high humidity may interfere with film drying.

Safelight Conditions

The purpose of safelighting is to provide enough illumination in the darkroom to allow the clinician to perform the processing procedures without compromising image quality. Safelight lamps are equipped with filters that eliminate the spectrum of white light to which the film is most sensitive, primarily green and blue light (Fig. 7–1). The filters permit passage of orange and red light to which film is less sensitive. The type of safelight filter to use

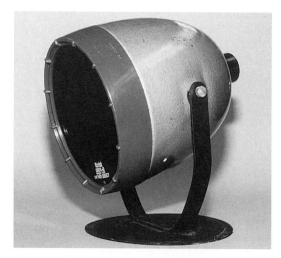

Figure 7–1. A darkroom safelight lamp, such as the one shown here, is equipped with a filter that eliminates the spectrum of white to which film is most sensitive.

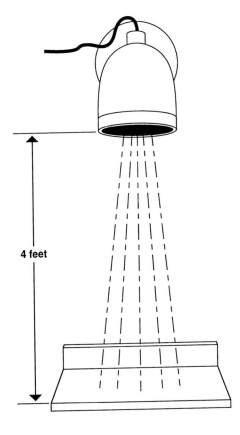

Figure 7–2. The safelight lamp should be mounted 4 feet from the work or counter surface where films will be handled in the darkroom.

4 feet

is an important consideration. The red filter is safe for both intraoral and extraoral radiographic film. The orange filter is safe for intraoral film. However, the orange filter is not safe for extraoral film and it will fog or slightly darken the overall image. Safelight filters should be free of cracks or scratches and correctly inserted into the lamp in order to eliminate white light leaks.

Radiographic film can be adversely affected if certain safelighting standards are not implemented. For intraoral and extraoral radiographic film, a 15-watt incandescent bulb should be used in the lamp. The lamp is mounted 4 feet from the work surface where films will be handled (Fig. 7–2). Several lamps may be needed to illuminate the darkroom adequately. For an indirect safelight lamp, one that is directed toward the ceiling, a 25-watt bulb should be used. The working time under safelight conditions is relatively short, approximately 5 minutes. Prolonged exposure of film to safelight will eventually result in film fog.

Darkroom Equipment

There are two types of processing systems, automatic and manual. In automatic processing, unwrapped films are guided through the developer, fixer, wash water, and dryer compartments of the machine via a series of rollers. In manual processing, the unwrapped films are placed on racks and moved through the developer, rinse water, fixer, wash water, and dryer by hand. Automatic processing systems have nearly replaced manual film processing because of their convenience, consistent performance, and reduced space requirements. However, their performance depends on frequent solution change and a strict regimen of machine cleaning and maintenance. Manual processing systems provide a good back-up method of film processing in the event of automated equipment breakdown.

The darkroom should be equipped with hot and cold running water and a sink facility for cleaning procedures and hand washing. Most automatic processors need only cold water, but water requirements do vary among processors. Adequate work space for film and cassette handling as well as storage space for chemicals, cassettes, and other materials should be provided. Manual processing systems require additional equipment, including a mixing valve (to regulate the incoming water temperature), solution tanks, solution stirrers, film racks, a floating thermometer, a timer, a film-drying rack, and a film dryer (Fig. 7–3).

Frequently, duplicate radiographs are needed for patient referrals or to reproduce records for patients who have relocated. A film duplicator should be considered a component of a well-equipped darkroom.

PROCESSING SYSTEMS

Several steps are involved in film processing: wetting, development, rinsing, fixing, washing, and drying. **Wetting** occurs during the first several seconds of developer solution contact with the film. Wetting softens the film emulsion so that the developer chemicals can act on the silver halide crystals. **Development** of the film transforms the latent image into the visible image by reduction of the exposed silver halide crystals into metallic silver. **Rinsing** stops film development and removes the excess chemicals from the emulsion. **Fixing** of the film removes the unexposed silver halide crystals from the emulsion, which produces clear zones on the film. In addition, the fixer

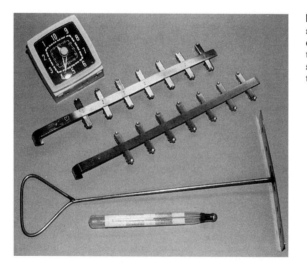

Figure 7–3. Manual processing systems require additional darkroom equipment, such as a timer, film-processing racks, a solution stir rod, and a thermometer.

solution hardens the film emulsion. **Washing** removes all excess chemicals from the film emulsion so that remnant fixer solution does not discolor the finished radiograph. Finally, **drying** of the processed film removes the water from the emulsion and prepares it for film mounting and viewing.

PROCESSING SOLUTIONS

Developer Solution

The developer solution has four components: developer, activator, restrainer, and preservative. Each constituent performs a particular function during image processing. The primary function of the developer solution is to transform the latent image into a visible image.

Developer. The developer or reducing agents, hydroquinone and metol, convert the exposed silver halide crystals into black metallic silver. Hydroquinone generates the black tones and contrast in the image, whereas metol is responsible for the gray tones. Phenidone replaces metol in automatic processing solutions but performs the same function.

Activator. Sodium carbonate is the activator agent in developer solution. It softens and swells the emulsion so that the reducing agents can act on the crystals more effectively. This chemical provides the alkaline environment needed for the reducing agents.

Restrainer. Potassium bromide restricts the reducing agents from developing the unexposed silver halide crystals. This prevents fog and the production of a dull, gray image that lacks contrast.

Preservative. The preservative agent is sodium sulfite. It prevents rapid oxidation and prolongs the life span of the reducing agents.

Solvent. Water is the medium into which the developer chemicals are dissolved.

Fixer Solution

The fixer solution also contains four components: fixing agent, acidifier, hardener, and preservative. The primary function of the fixer is to remove the undeveloped silver halide crystals from the film emulsion, thus clearing the film.

Fixing Agent. The fixing, or clearing, agent is sodium or ammonium thiosulfate ("hypo"). This chemical dissolves the unexposed, undeveloped silver halide crystals from the emulsion.

Acidifier. Acetic or sulfuric acid serves to neutralize any alkali carried over from the developer solution into the fixer solution. It terminates film development and provides the acidic environment necessary for fixation.

Hardener. The hardening agent, aluminum chloride or aluminum sulfide, shrinks and hardens the softened, swollen emulsion. The hardening agent helps the emulsion become damage resistant and reduces the film drying time.

Preservative. As in the developer solution, the preservative agent is sodium sulfite. It prevents chemical deterioration of the fixing solution.

Solvent. Water is the medium into which the fixer chemicals are dissolved.

Solution Replenishment

Processing chemicals lose their effectiveness and become exhausted with use, exposure to air, and contamination with water or other processing chemicals. Continued use without refortifying the solutions will result in poor quality films. To ensure optimal solution performance and high-quality radiographs, the chemicals should be replenished on a daily basis. Replenishing solutions restore the ability of the chemicals to perform their functions without changing the entire volume of solution. Replenishing solutions are available as ready-to-use developer or fixer solutions, or in the concentrated form of each solution. Replenished solutions should be replaced with fresh solutions every 3 to 4 weeks under normal conditions or more frequently when indicated.

AUTOMATIC FILM PROCESSING

Most automatic processors (Fig. 7–4) are constructed with a transport system that consists of a series of rollers driven by a constant speed motor operating via gears, belts, or chains. Usually the rollers are independent assemblies, one for each step in the processing sequence. The rollers guide the unwrapped films through the various solution compartments (developer, fixer, wash) and a blow dryer prior to their exit from the system (Fig. 7–5). The rollers perform several functions in addition to film transport. They massage and uniformly distribute the chemicals over the film, which speeds development and fixation. And they act as a squeegee, which removes the chemicals and water from the film emulsion and reduces chemical carryover into the fixer solution and wash water. This is an especially important function because there is no rinse cycle between developer and fixer solutions. Because of the roller contact with the film, both a hardening agent and an antiswelling agent are added to automatic developer solution, and an additional hardener is added to the fixer solution to prevent the emulsion from sticking to the rollers and being removed from the film base.

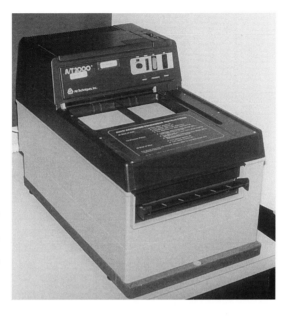

Figure 7–4. This is a typical example of an automatic processor. The on/off switch, time display, and temperature display are located on the upper right-hand corner of the machine. The film insertion tray is shown in the foreground and the film exit tray is located below the top control panel.

The average automatic processing time is approximately 5 minutes. This short time interval is the result of processing the films at higher temperatures, usually in the range of 85°F (29°C) to 105°F (40°C). Automatic processors contain a heating element that controls the temperature of the developer solution. The rollers are designed to rotate at a speed compatible with the temperature of the developer solution. Thus, the speed of the rollers as well as the processing time can be adjusted by altering the temperature of the developer solution. Time and temperature are inversely proportional. The processing time decreases as the temperature increases and vice versa. To produce high-quality radiographs, the optimum time and temperature settings recommended by the manufacturer should be followed.

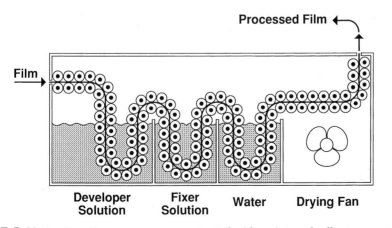

Figure 7–5. Most automatic processors are constructed with an internal roller transport system. The rollers guide the unwrapped films through the developer solution, fixer solution, water bath, and blow dryer prior to exiting the system.

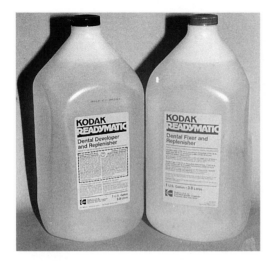

Figure 7–6. Automatic processing systems require specially formulated solutions that are compatible with the transport system, elevated temperatures, and lack of rinsing between developer and fixer solutions. Ready-to-use chemicals are convenient and time-saving.

Automatic processing systems require specially formulated solutions that are compatible with the mechanical transport system, higher temperatures, and lack of film rinsing between developer and fixer solutions. Most chemical and replenisher solutions are available either in concentrated or ready-to-use forms (Fig. 7–6). The concentrated formulation requires dilution with water.

Darkroom Film-Processing Procedures

The film packets should be handled in accordance with the infection control guidelines discussed in Chapter 6. Conventional darkrooms permit use of the film drop-out technique to prepare the films for processing. The basic procedures are as follows:

1. Wear fresh gloves to enter the darkroom, set out clean paper towels, set down the film receptacle, and handle the contaminated films.

2. In safelight conditions, remove the outer wrapping and lead foil, and drop out each film from between the black inner paper onto a fresh paper towel. Avoid contact with the film.

3. Once all the films have been dropped out, discard the contaminated wrappings.

4. Remove and dispose of the contaminated gloves; wash and dry the hands.

5. Handle each film on the edges. Place the film onto the intake mechanism and feed it into the processor. Most models allow several films to be fed simultaneously (Fig. 7–7). Care must be taken to allow ample space between each inserted film as well as between subsequent films.

6. Retrieve the finished films from the outlet tray or receptacle.

Daylight Loader Film-Processing Procedures

The film packets should be handled in accordance with the infection control guidelines discussed in Chapter 6. Daylight loader automatic processors (Fig.

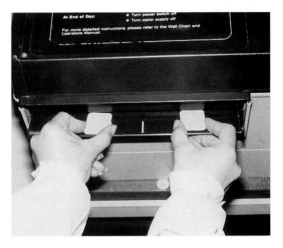

Figure 7–7. Once the films have been dropped out of the packets, they can be handled on the edges with clean, dry hands. The films should be inserted into the film intake mechanism with ample space between films.

7–8) require the use of the barrier film drop-out technique or the film immersion technique to prepare the films for processing. The basic procedures are as follows:

1. Place the prepared films into a disposable cup or onto a fresh paper towel.

2. Prepare the daylight loader box by placing plastic wrap or paper toweling over the bottom inner surface of the unit.

3. Place the film receptacle and powderless gloves inside the unit and close the lid.

4. Insert clean hands through the sleeve portals and don the gloves.

Figure 7–8. Daylight loader automatic processors, like the one pictured here, require special film handling techniques and daylight loader box preparation prior to film processing to prevent microbial contamination of the unit.

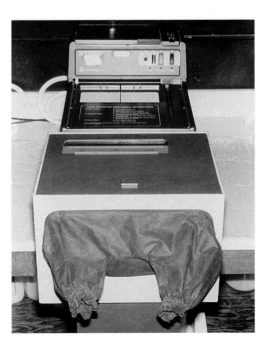

5. Shell the films, handle each film on the edges, and insert the films into the feed mechanism as previously described (see Figure 7–7).

6. When all films have been inserted, remove the gloves and withdraw the hands.

7. Open the daylight loader lid, enfold the waste into the bottom covering materials, and remove and discard them.

PRECAUTIONARY MEASURES

Several film-handling methods must be avoided to prevent automatic film processing errors and processor malfunctioning. If the film edges were bent during exposure procedures, they must be unbent prior to insertion. Otherwise, they may get caught in the rollers or diverted into the solution reservoirs. If films are fed too quickly with inadequate spacing, they will become stuck together during processing or get caught in the roller system. Unsightly artifacts are the result. Finally, previously processed or incompletely processed damp or wet films should not be re-fed into the machine, as this will contaminate the solutions and rollers as well as produce streaking on subsequent films.

AUTOMATIC PROCESSOR MAINTENANCE

Automatic processing systems require a strict regimen of solution replenishment, unit and roller cleaning, solution change, and maintenance of the moving parts. Automatic processor performance depends on completion of these procedures. Routine maintenance will help prevent unit breakdown and a myriad of processing problems and errors.

Replenishment

Automatic processing solutions should be replenished daily, and more frequently when indicated. After processing the equivalent of four full mouth surveys or panoramic films, 4 to 6 ounces of processing chemicals should be added to each solution. This ensures that the chemicals are of adequate concentration and level to perform their tasks. Some systems have an automatic replenisher mechanism in which the solution reservoirs are connected via hoses to the developer and fixer tanks. When activated, these mechanisms supply the chemicals needed to replenish each solution. Otherwise, replenishment must be done by hand. Failure to do so will result in poor quality films.

Roller Care

The rollers are cleaned daily by running a cleaning sheet, a clear piece of film base material, through the roller system (Fig. 7–9). This procedure helps remove foreign debris and residual gelatin from the rollers. Reuse of the

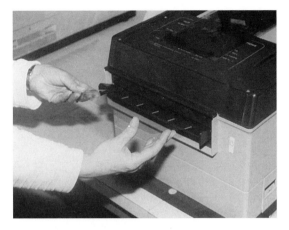

Figure 7–9. The automatic processor roller transport system should be cleaned daily by sending a cleaning sheet through the system. This removes foreign debris and residual gelatin from the rollers.

cleaning sheets is not recommended because of possible solution contamination. In addition, the rollers are removed from the processor and cleaned on a weekly basis. As a precaution, the operator wears a protective gown, utility gloves, a mask, and eyewear when performing the weekly roller-cleaning procedures. The rollers are rinsed under warm running water. A special cleaning solution or a mild, nonabrasive cleaner is sprayed or applied to the rinsed rollers and allowed to sit for 10 minutes. Then, the roller system is wiped with a sponge or cleaned with a nonabrasive brush (a separate sponge or brush for each roller assembly to avoid solution contamination) while the operator turns the gear mechanisms by hand. Each assembly is thoroughly rinsed and excess water removed before reinstallation into the processor. Generally speaking, soaking rollers in water for a period of time is an ineffective means of cleaning or rinsing the transport system.

Solution Change

Replenished solutions are replaced with fresh solutions every 2 to 4 weeks under normal conditions. Manufacturers of automated nonroller transport system processors recommend that all solutions be changed every 2 weeks. The processor is thoroughly cleaned at each solution change (Fig. 7–10). The operator wears a protective gown, utility gloves, a mask, and eyewear when cleaning the entire processing system. The processor compartments are drained and cleaned with a commercial cleaner, warm water, and separate sponges or nonabrasive brushes. The rollers are cleaned as previously described. The compartments and rollers are thoroughly rinsed with warm water prior to reassembly. Periodically (once every 3 months), a systems cleaner can be used to clean hard-to-reach areas more thoroughly. After its use, the system should be rinsed several times to remove all traces of the cleaner chemicals. Residual system cleaner chemicals will contaminate the processing solutions.

When replacing the chemicals, always fill the fixer reservoir first. As a precaution, rinse the developer reservoir just in case of a fixer splash during

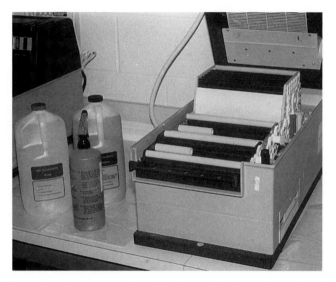

Figure 7–10. The automatic processor should be thoroughly cleaned at each solution change. The compartments and rollers should be cleaned with a commercial cleaner, warm water, and separate sponges or nonabrasive brushes.

filling of the fixer reservoir. Even a few droplets of fixer can contaminate the developer solution, requiring replacement with fresh chemicals.

Monthly Maintenance

Once a month, inspect the moving parts (rollers, gears, turning mechanism) for wear and lubricate, as needed, prior to reassembly. Check the dryer and remove any accumulated dust.

Daily Routine

At the beginning of the day, replenish the solutions and allow the solutions to reach their optimum temperature. To clean the rollers, send a "cleaning sheet" through the roller transport system. At the end of the day, remove the main cover or prop it open to allow the chemical fumes to escape. This prevents condensation from forming underneath the unit cover, which may drip back into the solutions, resulting in contamination.

MANUAL FILM PROCESSING

Manual processing requires the use of hot and cold running water, regulated by a mixing valve, and a master water tank into which developer and fixer reservoirs are inserted (Fig. 7–11). The master water tank temperature should be maintained at 68°F (20°C) to 70°F (21°C) to provide an optimal solution processing temperature. Customarily, the developer is inserted into

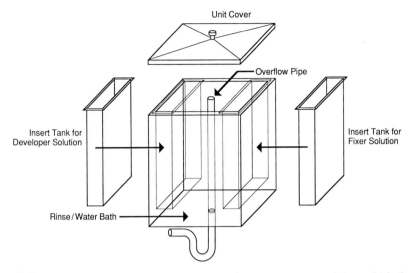

Figure 7–11. A manual processing system consists of a master water tank into which the developer and fixer solution tanks are inserted. The water bath should have an overflow pipe to allow a constant exchange of fresh circulating water.

the left side of the master tank and the fixer on the right side. The water bath between the developer and fixer reservoirs serves as the rinse and wash baths during film processing (Fig. 7–12). The water bath should have an overflow pipe to allow a constant exchange of fresh, running water. This prevents chemical contamination of the water bath during film rinsing and washing. A floating thermometer is inserted into the water bath to allow periodic temperature checks (see Figure 7–3).

As with automatic processing, time and temperature are inversely proportional. The processing time decreases as the temperature increases and vice

Figure 7–12. A standard manual processing tank is shown here with the solution reservoirs inserted into the master tank and the overflow pipe in the water bath.

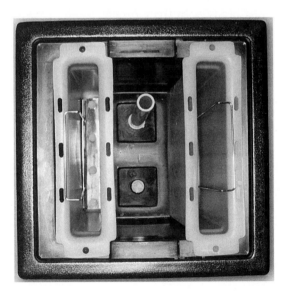

Table 7-1. Developer Temperature and Time

Temperature (°F)	Time (Minutes)
65	6
68	5
70	4.5
72	4
76	3

versa. To produce high-quality radiographs, the films are processed in the developer for 4.5 to 5 minutes at 68°F (20°C) to 70°F (21°C), rinsed 20 to 30 seconds, fixed 9 to 10 minutes, and washed 20 minutes. The time of processing can be monitored by use of an interval timer (see Figure 7–3). For fluctuations in temperature, refer to the guidelines in Table 7–1.

Processing films at extreme darkroom temperatures will reduce film contrast and increase film fog.

Manual Film-Processing Procedures

Many steps are involved in the manual processing of exposed films. Attention to each detail will help ensure high-quality film results. The overall processing time at the optimum temperature ranges from 45 to 60 minutes if commercial film dryers are used.

Prior to beginning film-processing procedures, the water is turned on and the solution temperature stabilized at the optimum processing temperature. The master tank cover is removed, the solutions replenished, and the solutions brought to their proper levels. Finally, the solutions are stirred with a plastic or stainless steel rod (separate rod for each solution) to make the temperature and concentration uniform (see Figure 7–3). Once these tasks are completed, the films can be prepared for processing using the film drop-out technique.

1. Wear fresh gloves to enter the darkroom, set out clean paper towels, set down the film receptacle, and handle the contaminated films.

2. Label the processing rack with the patient's name as well as survey date.

3. In safelight conditions, remove the outer wrapping and lead foil, and drop out each film from between the black inner paper onto a fresh paper towel. Avoid contact with the film.

4. Once all the films have been dropped out, discard the contaminated wrappings.

5. Remove and dispose of the contaminated gloves; wash and dry the hands.

6. Handle each film on the edges and attach each film to the processing

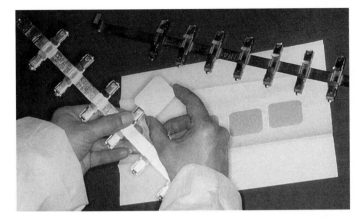

Figure 7–13. Once the films have been dropped out of the packets, they can be handled on the edges with clean, dry hands. The films should be attached to the processing rack with adequate space between films.

rack (Fig. 7–13). Leave enough space between the films so that they do not overlap.

7. Insert the films with slight agitation into the developer solution and set the timer for the proper interval. If the clinician intends to leave the darkroom, the tanks must be covered with the master tank lid during the development cycle.

8. After the development time has expired, immediately remove the films from the developer. Place them into the water bath, agitate, and rinse for 20 to 30 seconds.

9. Immerse the films with slight agitation into the fixer solution and set the timer for 10 minutes. If the clinician intends to leave the darkroom, the tanks must be covered with the master tank lid. If the films need to be viewed immediately, the films can be removed and rinsed after 3 minutes. After inspection, the films must be returned to the fixer solution to complete the cycle for the remaining 7 minutes.

10. After 10 minutes, the films can be transferred from the fixer solution to the water bath. The films should wash for 20 minutes to remove all residual chemicals. Films should not be washed overnight as the film emulsion will slide off the film base with such a prolonged washing cycle.

11. After 20 minutes, remove the films from the water bath and shake off the excess water. The films can be placed in a commercial dryer to expedite film drying. If the films are left to air dry, they are hung on a towel rack over a drip pan until completely dry.

At the end of the day, turn off the water and cover the processing tanks.

MANUAL PROCESSING MAINTENANCE

Manual processing systems require fresh or replenisher chemicals designed for manual processing. Automatic processing chemicals cannot be used for manual processing.

Replenishment

The developer and fixer solutions are replenished daily with 8 ounces of an appropriate replenisher, even if no films were processed. This may require removal of enough solution from each tank to add the replenisher. The level of the solution should be adequate enough to cover all the films attached to the processing rack. Replenished solutions are replaced with fresh chemicals every 3 to 4 weeks.

Solution Change

With manual processing systems, the solution reservoirs and master processing tank need to be thoroughly cleaned at each solution change. When performing these cleaning procedures, the operator wears a protective gown, utility gloves, a mask, and eyewear. The solution reservoirs and water bath are drained and cleaned with a commercial cleaner or mild cleaning agent, warm water, and separate sponges or brushes. The master and solution tanks are thoroughly rinsed with water before reassembly and solution replacement. Developer and fixer reservoirs should not be exchanged due to the possible solution contamination with residual chemicals. The fixer tank is filled first to avoid contamination of the developer solution. The solutions are stirred after filling and prior to film processing.

WASTE MANAGEMENT

The federal Resource Conservation and Recovery Act (RCRA) of 1976 was enacted to prevent environmental damage from discarded waste materials. In most areas of the United States, the average-sized dental office is classified by the RCRA agency as a "Conditionally Exempt Small Quantity Generator." Because of the small volume of hazardous waste produced, most dental offices are exempt from the majority of federal hazardous waste regulations. However, some states and local agencies require that any amount of hazardous waste be disposed of according to regulations. Therefore, it is paramount for every dental office and clinic to be familiar and in compliance with current disposal regulations in their community.

The most typical means of managing radiographic wastes generated in the dental office is to discard them in the trash or pour them down the drain. However, some wastes, such as fixer solution, which contains silver, and the lead foil from the film packet, are identified by the RCRA as hazardous or regulated by other agencies that control effluent disposal into municipal sewer systems or septic tank systems.

There are several methods for properly disposing of the silver and lead foil. Silver can be recovered from fixer solutions by metallic replacement or electroplating procedures. The metallic replacement method utilizes a chemical recovery cartridge through which the waste solution is poured. Within the cartridge, the silver reacts with iron to form a silver sludge while the iron goes into solution. Electroplating requires the effluent to pass between two electrodes through which a direct current flows. The silver plates out on the cathode electrode.

The lead foil should be separated from the film wrappings after processing and disposed of according to federal, state, or local regulations. If the lead foil is not separated from the other film wrappings, the waste could be considered hazardous under RCRA regulations and require management as a hazardous waste. These wastes can be properly managed by a waste disposal company. Such companies are licensed to pick up waste materials and dispose of them according to federal, state, or local regulations as well as provide documentation of the disposal.

HAZARD COMMUNICATION STANDARD

The Occupational Safety and Health Administration's (OSHA) Hazard Communication Standard was adopted to reduce chemically related occupational illnesses and injuries. The Standard assists employers in formulating a comprehensive hazard communication program, which includes a written office or clinic manual, container labeling, other forms of warning, material safety data sheets (MSDS), and employee training. It is the responsibility of the employer to inform employees of all safety materials provided, required personal protective devices, and safe handling and disposal methods.

The hazardous chemicals in the Standard are limited to those present in the workplace to which employees may be exposed under normal working conditions and in the case of a possible emergency. Material safety data sheets should be obtained for all chemicals in the workplace and be readily accessible to employees. The MSDS contain product information such as chemical composition, hazardous ingredients, health and safety hazards, spill or leak procedures, and precautions for safe handling, use, and disposal. MSDS can be obtained from the chemical manufacturer or importer, or from the American Dental Association.

IMAGE TRANSFORMATION

The radiographic film emulsion consists of a homogeneous mixture of silver halide crystals and gelatin. The emulsion is coated onto each side of the transparent plastic film base. Each silver halide crystal is a lattice of mostly silver (Ag^+) and bromide (Br^-) ions, and small amounts of iodide (I^-) ions (Fig. 7–14A). The shape and lattice structure of the crystal are not perfect. Some of the imperfections result in the imaging property of the crystal called the sensitivity speck (Fig. 7–14A). During film processing, silver atoms tend to be attracted to and concentrate at the site of the sensitivity speck. Each crystal has many such imperfections or sensitivity specks. In the silver halide crystal, both atoms and ions are free to migrate within the crystal. The halide ions concentrate along the surface of the crystal while the silver ions tend to aggregate inside the crystal. The sensitivity speck is thought to be located on or near the surface of the crystal.

When an x-ray photon interacts with the silver halide crystal, a secondary electron is released either by photoelectric or Compton interaction. The sec-

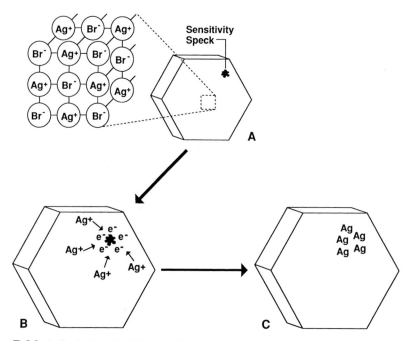

Figure 7-14. *A,* Each silver halide crystal is a lattice of mostly silver (Ag+) and bromide (Br−) ions. Imperfections in the shape and lattice structure of the crystal form the sensitivity speck. *B,* Migrating electrons (e−) are attracted to the sensitivity speck and impart a negative charge to the region. As a result, silver (Ag+) ions are attracted to the negative charge of the sensitivity speck. *C,* The silver ions are neutralized and converted into metallic silver, which forms the latent image center. (Adapted from Miles DA, Van Dis ML, Razmus TF: Basic Principles of Oral and Maxillofacial Radiology. Philadelphia, WB Saunders, 1992, p 156.)

ondary electron is released with sufficient energy to travel a large distance in the crystal and may dislodge additional electrons from the crystal lattice. As a result, a number of electrons are released and travel through the lattice. Some of the migrating electrons become trapped in the area of the sensitivity speck and impart a negative charge to the region. As the halide ions that lost their electrons become neutral and move out of the crystal into the gelatin, the positively charged silver ions are attracted to the negative charge of the sensitivity speck (Fig. 7–14B). After the silver ions reach the area of the sensitivity speck, they are neutralized and converted into atoms of metallic silver. The aggregate of metallic silver atoms is called the latent image center (Fig. 7–14C). The crystals with latent image centers constitute the latent image. It is the metallic silver or latent image center that makes the crystals sensitive to development and formation of the visible image. The developer solution converts the metallic silver deposited at the latent image center into black, metallic silver grains. The fixer removes the unexposed, undeveloped silver bromide crystals and clears the film in those areas. The black, metallic silver grains that remain in the gelatin form the visible image.

FILM MOUNTING

Processed intraoral radiographs should be placed in a specially designed frame for convenient viewing and storage. The mounted films are organized anatomically and in a sequential manner, which facilitates correlation with the patient's oral cavity and interpretation of the radiographs.

Opaque pocket mounts are recommended for mounting intraoral radiographs. The clear plastic pockets or windows in the frame provide protection for the films while the opaque frame material blocks out extraneous light around the film windows. The number and arrangement of the film windows should match the number and orientation of the radiographs.

Types of Film Mounting

There are two basic methods of film mounting, labial and lingual. Labial mounting positions the convexity (raised bump) of the film identification dot toward the viewer. The films are organized and mounted as if the viewer were looking at the patient's face. This arrangement places the patient's right side on the viewer's left. Labial mounting is the preferred method and is advocated by the American Dental Association. Lingual mounting positions the concavity (depression) of the film identification dot toward the viewer. The films are organized and mounted as if the viewer were sitting on the patient's tongue looking out. This arrangement places the patient's right side on the viewer's right side.

Film-Mounting Procedures

The finished radiographs can be efficiently organized on a clean, flat viewbox surface (Fig. 7–15). This permits viewing of each image while arranging the films into proper order. The films should be handled on the edges with clean, dry hands. The following guidelines will assist the viewer in mounting intraoral periapicals and bitewings.

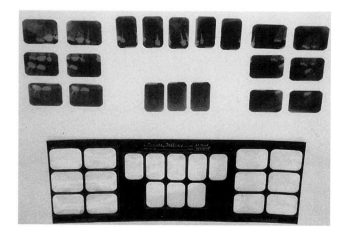

Figure 7–15. The finished radiographs can be efficiently organized on a clean, flat viewbox surface. This permits viewing of each image while arranging the films into proper order.

1. Select an appropriate film mount and label it with the patient's name and date of the films.

2. Place all films on the viewbox surface with the convexity of the film identification dot in an upward direction.

3. Locate and arrange the bitewing radiographs. The plane of occlusion should form a smile configuration, and the teeth crowns should appear in their proper order.

4. Identify and arrange the vertical anterior periapicals, beginning with the central incisor views. Then place the adjacent lateral incisor and canine views into their respective positions relative to the central incisor views.

5. Locate and arrange the horizontal posterior periapicals and match the crowns of the teeth on the periapicals with the crowns on the bitewing films.

6. After all the films have been arranged, review the organized films with respect to the normal sequence of the teeth, tooth morphology, and anatomical landmarks. Make any necessary corrections.

7. Transfer the correctly arranged radiographs into the film-mounting frame. Check the mounted survey to be sure that the films were placed in the proper windows.

FILM DUPLICATION

On occasion it is necessary to copy or duplicate radiographs for the purposes of patient referral, record transfer, or third party requests. The duplication of radiographs provides a means of producing additional copies of a survey while maintaining the original films.

One method of creating a duplicate set of radiographs is by using double film packets for intraoral imaging. Double film packets produce two films with one exposure. The two films must be separated prior to insertion into the automatic processor or being attached to the manual film-processing racks.

The most common method of film duplication requires the use of a film duplicator and duplication film (Fig. 7–16). With this method, ultraviolet light is transmitted through the original survey, which exposes the specially designed duplication film. The exposed film is processed as usual by either an automatic or a manual processing system. Commercial film duplicators provide an ultraviolet light source, a timer for the light exposure, and a lid with a closing mechanism. Duplication film is a single emulsion film that is particularly sensitive to ultraviolet light. Unlike x-ray film, duplication film produces a positive image. The areas exposed to light become clear when processed rather than dark. Duplication film is available in many sizes, including a periapical film size.

Film duplication procedures must be completed in the darkroom in safelight conditions. Close contact between the original survey and the duplication film is necessary to avoid blurred images on the duplicate film. Thin, flat pocket mounts are recommended for organizing intraoral radiographs for duplication procedures. Duplication film, with the exception of the periapical size, does not have film identification dots. Therefore, duplicated surveys should always be referenced with the original survey to identify the patient's right and left sides correctly and to label the survey with the patient's name and survey date (Fig. 7–17).

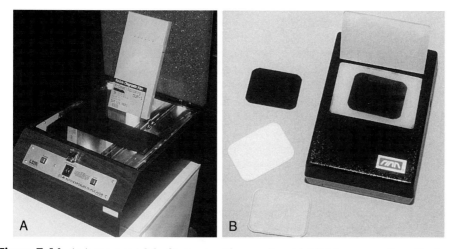

Figure 7-16. *A*, A commercial duplicator provides an ultraviolet light source, a timer for the light exposure, and a lid with a closing mechanism. The mounted survey is placed toward the light source, and the emulsion side of the duplication film is placed against the rear surface of the survey mount. *B*, A small, handheld duplicator can be used to duplicate a single periapical or bitewing film.

Film duplication has another advantage. High- or low-density radiographs can be improved by film duplication. Often, it provides a means of salvaging films that, under normal circumstances, must be retaken.

Duplication Procedures

The following guidelines provide a step-by-step approach to film duplication. The procedure begins with correctly mounted intraoral radiographs or a properly oriented extraoral film.

1. Evaluate the film density of the survey to determine the amount of light needed to duplicate it. High-density radiographs require more light exposure, whereas low-density radiographs require less light exposure. The light

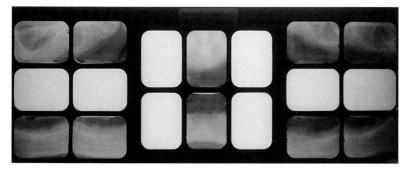

Figure 7-17. The duplicated survey should be referenced with the original survey to identify correctly the patient's right and left sides and to label the survey with the patient's name and the survey date. A duplicated periapical edentulous survey is pictured.

exposure can be adjusted relative to the light exposure recommended by the duplicator's manufacturer for films of normal film density.

2. Place the mounted survey or extraoral film with the viewing surface (dot convexities) toward the light source of the duplicator. Set the exposure timer.

3. In safelight conditions, remove a sheet of duplication film from its storage box. The emulsion side of the film can be identified by its dull, light-colored appearance in comparison with the shiny, dark-colored nonemulsion side.

4. Place the emulsion side of the film against the rear surface of the film or mount and center it over the survey.

5. Close the duplicator lid and fasten the closing device. This presses the duplication film against the original survey and light source, which provides the close contact necessary for quality results.

6. Press the timer button to expose the duplication film to light.

7. Open the lid, remove the film, and process the film as usual.

8. Evaluate the density and quality of the duplicated film. If the image is too dark, the light exposure should be increased. If the image is too light, the light exposure should be decreased. Repeat the procedure if the image is not acceptable.

9. Reference the duplicate film with the original survey to determine the patient's right and left side and to label it with the patient's name and the date of the survey.

QUALITY ASSURANCE

Radiographic quality assurance is a plan of action employed to ensure that high-quality, diagnostic images are produced while minimizing costs and radiation exposure to patients and personnel. Quality assurance is achieved through regular testing, planned monitoring, and scheduled maintenance. Frequently, quality assurance tasks are delegated to supporting personnel, but the dentist is ultimately responsible for quality assurance in his or her office. The quality assurance program rationale and tasks should be discussed with the supporting personnel. For the program to be successful, the tasks and the specific persons responsible for completing the tasks should be clearly outlined, preferably in written form.

The components of a radiographic quality control program include performance testing and maintenance of the x-ray equipment, darkroom conditions, processing systems, image receptors, and viewing conditions. In addition, the technical expertise of the radiographer should be reviewed periodically to assure that retakes are kept to a minimum. This can be accomplished by maintaining a retake log that details the number of retakes, the type of errors committed, and the radiographer responsible for the errors.

X-Ray Equipment

Periodic evaluation and calibration of the x-ray machine promotes consistent performance and reduces re-exposures due to equipment malfunctions. Annually, the x-ray unit should be tested for x-ray output, kilovoltage calibration, half value layer, timer accuracy, milliamperage reproducibility, collimation, beam alignment, and tube head stability (see Chapter 2). These tests can be performed by the dentist but require some basic testing devices and materials. The tests can also be completed by the equipment manufacturer's service representative. In either case, the specific tests and their results should be documented in a log book. X-ray machine testing and inspection are often regulated by a state agency, and the frequency of the inspection varies according to state regulations.

Darkroom Conditions

White leaks around doorframes, ceiling tiles, vents, and wall seams should be eliminated with black tape or weatherstripping. To detect and eliminate white light leaks, enter the darkroom, close the door, turn off all the lights, allow the eyes to adjust to the dark for several minutes, look for light leaks, and mark them with white chalk. Seal the leaks as previously described. Another test for white light leaks is called the coin test (Fig. 7–18). With all the darkroom lights out, place a coin onto the surface of an unwrapped film and let it remain in place for 5 minutes. After 5 minutes, turn on the safelight and process the film. If an image of the coin is visible on the processed film, white light leaks are present and need to be eliminated (Fig. 7–19).

The filter, bulb, and distance requirements for safelighting have been presented. Periodically, filters should be checked for fading, cracks, or scratches. The coin test can be used to check safelight conditions, presuming that white light leaks have been eliminated (Fig. 7–18). In safelight conditions, place a coin onto the surface of an unwrapped film on the countertop where films are prepared for processing. Let it remain in place for 5 minutes, then process the film. If an image of the coin is visible on the processed film, the safelight conditions need to be re-evaluated and corrections made (Fig. 7–19). Daylight loader filters can also be evaluated with the coin test.

Processing Systems

One of the major causes of retakes is improper film-processing procedures. The processing systems should be cleaned and inspected regularly and the

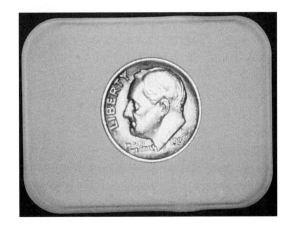

Figure 7-18. The coin test can be used to check for white light leaks or proper safelight conditions. A coin is placed onto an unwrapped film for 5 minutes with the darkroom lights out or under safelight conditions. After 5 minutes, the film is processed.

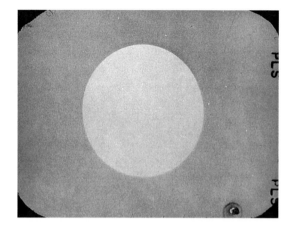

Figure 7-19. An image of the coin on the processed coin test film indicates white light leaks or improper safelight conditions.

solutions replenished and changed as previously discussed. The best way to eliminate processing problems and the resultant retakes is to monitor the processing solutions on a daily basis. This can be done by producing a control or reference film and a check or monitor film with a stepwedge. A stepwedge is a device with graduated thicknesses of metal (usually aluminum or copper), similar to the configuration of a staircase. When an exposure is made of a stepwedge placed between the x-ray source and a film, various degrees of densities are recorded and made visible on the processed film. A stepwedge device can be purchased commercially or constructed by hand with lead foils from intraoral film packets (Fig. 7–20). A lead foil stepwedge can be created by stacking varying thicknesses of lead foils on top of each other in a staircase fashion. Each layer can be increased by one lead foil thickness until several increments form the stepwedge. The stepwedge can be held together with tape. Control and checker films can also be produced with an inexpensive commercial test tool device (Fig. 7–20).

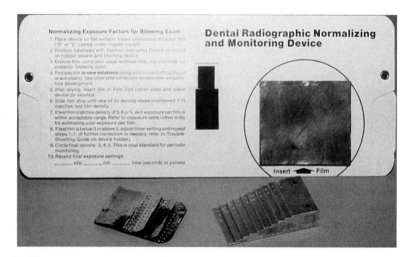

Figure 7-20. Processing solution control and check films can be produced with a number of test devices: an inexpensive commercial monitoring device, a commercial aluminum stepwedge, or a homemade lead foil stepwedge.

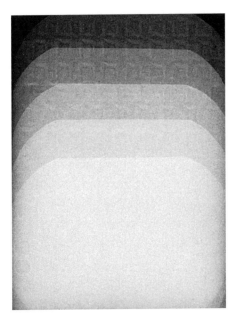

Figure 7–21. A control or reference film should be made at each solution change. The control film should be processed in fresh solutions, mounted in an opaque mount, and kept for reference until the solutions are changed.

Solution Monitoring

A control or reference radiograph is made at each solution change. A fresh, unexpired, properly stored film is used to produce the radiograph. Place the stepwedge on top of the film packet and expose it at a molar time setting, with the PID (position indicating device) directed perpendicular to both the stepwedge and film. The distance between the open end of the PID and the film should be minimal. It is essential that the same exposure and distance factors be used when producing the check or monitor film. The control film is processed in fresh solutions, mounted in an opaque mount, and kept on a viewbox for reference until solutions are changed (Fig. 7–21).

Prior to processing patient films each day, a check film is exposed in the same manner as described for the control film. After the solutions are replenished and the optimum solution temperature stabilized, the check film is processed (Fig. 7–22). The check film and the control film should appear identical. If there is a visible difference between the two films, there is a processing problem. The solutions may be exhausted, be contaminated, be too hot or too cold, or require additional replenishment or a solution change. The problem should be resolved before patient films are processed.

Image Receptors

Unexposed film should be kept in a cool, dry place away from any x-ray source or chemical fumes. Ideally, films should be stored at between 50°F (10°C) and 70°F (21°C) and between 30% and 50% relative humidity. Film should be used before its expiration date.

Periodically, cassettes used for extraoral radiography are inspected. Flexi-

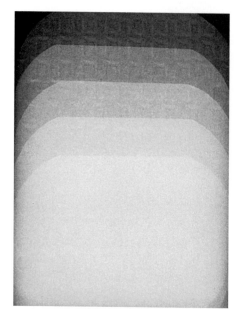

Figure 7–22. A check or monitor film should be made each day before patient films are processed. The film should be processed after replenishing the solutions and stabilizing the solution temperature. The control film and check film should appear identical. If there is a visible difference, a processing problem exists.

ble panoramic cassettes are examined for cracks around the seams and defects in the latch mechanism. Rigid cassettes are examined for defects in the latch mechanism and hinge device. Proper care of the intensifying screens is also important. The screens are inspected on a regular basis for cracks or defects in the screen surface. Defective screens should be replaced, because the defects will produce artifacts on the film. In addition, intensifying screens should be cleaned periodically with a special screen cleaner and antistatic solution. The screens are cleaned with a cotton ball or gauze square dampened with the cleaning agent (Fig. 7–23). After each screen is cleaned, it is wiped dry with a clean, dry cotton ball or gauze square, and the cassette is left open until the screens are completely dry.

Viewbox Care

The viewbox, an essential but often neglected piece of radiographic equipment, permits viewing and interpretation of the radiographs. The surface should be free of cracks, and the illumination should be even and not flicker. Burned out light bulbs should be replaced immediately. As presented in Chapter 6, the operatory viewbox is precleaned, disinfected, and covered to prevent aerosol contamination during invasive procedures. A mounted set of radiographs can be placed under the plastic cover for easy reference during intraoral procedures (Fig. 7–24). The nonoperatory viewbox is cleaned regularly to remove debris and dust from the surface that may interfere with radiographic interpretation (Fig. 7–25).

FILM HANDLING AND PROCESSING ARTIFACTS

Numerous errors can occur if the radiographer does NOT handle the film properly, maintain a clean darkroom environment, or implement and main-

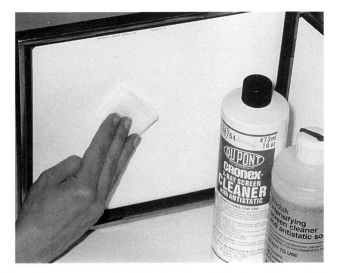

Figure 7–23. Intensifying screens should be cleaned periodically with a special screen cleaner and antistatic solution. The screens should be cleaned with a cotton ball or gauze square dampened with the cleaning solution. A fresh cotton ball or gauze square should be used to dry the clean screen surface.

tain high-quality processing standards. The most common problems include mishandling of the film, contamination of the emulsion with chemicals, underprocessing or overprocessing of the film, and improper film insertion or racking techniques. Many times the processed image is so compromised that it must be retaken.

Film-Handling Artifacts

A number of artifacts are produced when the film packet or the unwrapped film is not handled in an appropriate manner.

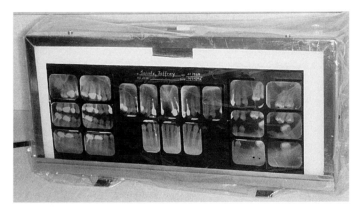

Figure 7–24. The operatory viewbox should be precleaned, disinfected, and covered to prevent aerosol contamination during invasive procedures. A mounted set of radiographs can be placed under the plastic cover for reference during intraoral procedures.

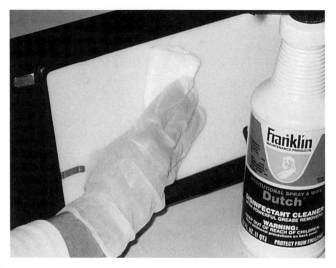

Figure 7–25. Viewboxes should be cleaned regularly to remove debris and dust from the glass surface that may interfere with radiographic interpretation.

Fingerprints

Black fingerprint marks are caused by handling the surface of the film with fingers contaminated with developer solution or fluoride (Fig. 7–26). To prevent these black fingerprint artifacts, the films should be handled on the edges with clean, dry hands. In addition, the darkroom environmental surfaces should be clean and free of chemical contaminates.

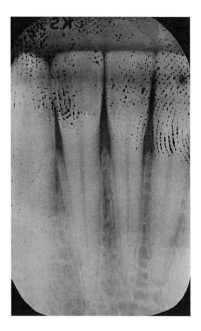

Figure 7–26. Fingerprint artifacts are caused by handling the film surface with fingers contaminated with developer solution or fluoride.

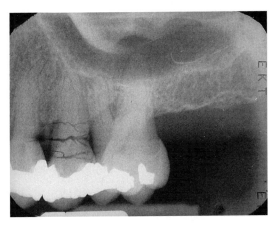

Figure 7–27. Static electricity produces branchlike artifacts on the processed film. Frequently, this error is caused by rough, rapid unwrapping of the film packet.

Static Electricity

Black lightning or branchlike artifacts on the processed film are caused by static electricity (Fig. 7–27). A dry office environment along with rough, rapid unwrapping of the film packet may produce static electricity. Synthetic uniform materials and rubber-soled shoes rubbing against carpet contribute to the generation of static electricity. To prevent static electricity artifacts, the film packet is opened slowly. The use of antistatic sprays on synthetic clothing will help reduce static electricity problems.

Scratched Emulsion

Careless handling of the film, especially during manual processing, often results in a scratched emulsion (Fig. 7–28). A white line or scratch occurs when a sharp object, such as a film rack or the clinician's fingernail, removes some of the softened film emulsion from the film base. A scratched emulsion can also occur during automatic processing if hardened deposits on the rollers scrape the film emulsion. Needless to say, care must be taken when placing

Figure 7–28. A white line or scratched emulsion occurs when a sharp object removes some of the softened film emulsion from the film base.

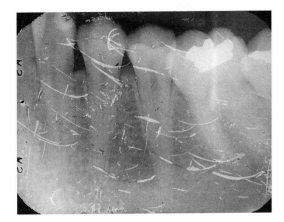

racks into the manual processing solutions, and automatic processor rollers must be clean and free of debris.

White Light Exposure

Radiographic film must be opened in safelight conditions. If the film packet is partially opened in white light, the exposed area will process black (Fig. 7–29). The portion of the film that remained protected by the wrapping materials will be unaffected. A film completely unwrapped in white light will be totally black when processed. With daylight loader automatic processing, the films must be fully inserted into the machine before the hands are withdrawn through the sleeve portals. In addition, the sleeve material must be tight fitting to seal out white light around the arms. Occasionally, white light leaks are the result of imperfections in the outer film wrapper or from rough handling of the packet during film placement and exposure procedures.

Fogged Image

A fogged film appears dull gray and lacks contrast and detail (Fig. 7–30). Film fog can be caused by a variety of factors: improper film storage, expired film, improper safelight conditions, white light leaks in the darkroom, contaminated processing solutions, or an elevated developer temperature. To prevent film fog, quality assurance measures should be implemented so that shortcomings can be identified and corrected.

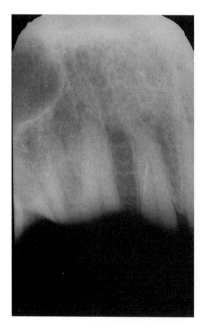

Figure 7–29. This film was partially exposed to white light. The coronal portion of the film that was exposed to white light appears black, while the apical portion of the film that remained protected appears normal.

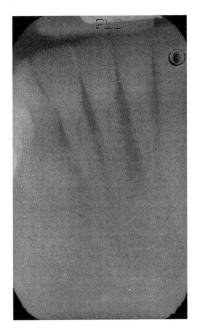

Figure 7–30. A fogged image has a dull, gray appearance and lacks contrast. Film fog can be caused by a number of problems: improper film storage, incorrect safelight conditions, white light leaks, or an elevated developer temperature.

Processing Errors and Artifacts

Poor quality radiographs and numerous artifacts can result from improper and careless processing techniques. Most problems can be easily identified and remedied with a quality assurance program and the radiographer's common sense.

Film-Feed Errors

When films are fed into the automatic processor too quickly or with inadequate spacing, the films become overlapped during film processing (Fig. 7–31). This can occur in manual processing as well when space is not provided

Figure 7–31. Films can become overlapped in the automatic processor when inserted too quickly or with inadequate space between films. The overlapped areas appear green when separated and darken with exposure to light.

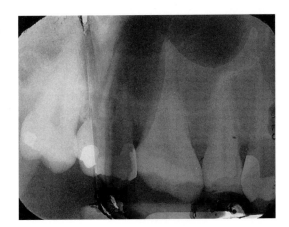

between films on the processing rack. The overlapped regions of the films are incompletely processed and, when separated, the green, underprocessed portions darken with exposure to white light. To remedy this problem, films must be fed into the automatic processor slowly and with adequate spacing or, in the case of manual processing, the films must be spaced adequately on the processing rack.

Torn Emulsion

Sometimes the emulsion is still wet or sticky after the automatic processing cycle is complete. Films can become stuck together and, upon separation, the emulsion can be torn from the film base (Fig. 7–32). In automatic processing, this may be the result of a faulty dryer, high humidity in the darkroom, low dryer or developer solution temperature, incorrect processing chemicals, or processing the film too quickly. These problems can be eliminated by following standard processing procedures and implementing quality assurance measures. In manual processing, this error usually occurs during the drying cycle when racks are positioned too close together, allowing surface contact between films.

Underdeveloped Film

An underdeveloped film has a light or low-density appearance (Fig. 7–33). It may be the result of inadequate development time, a cool developer temperature, or diluted, exhausted, or contaminated developer solution. Other possibilities include a faulty thermometer, timer, or automatic processor heating element. To prevent this error, the temperature of the solutions should be checked and the temperature and development time adjusted as needed. To check solution performance, a check film should be produced to determine whether the solutions need to be replenished or changed. Finally, any faulty equipment should be replaced.

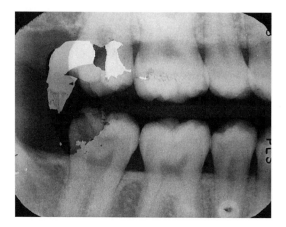

Figure 7–32. Sometimes the emulsion is not completely dry after automatic film processing, and films may become stuck together. When the films are separated, the emulsion can be torn from the film base, as seen on the maxillary second molar crown of this bitewing film.

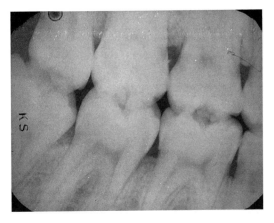

Figure 7–33. An underprocessed image has a light, or low-density, appearance. It may be the result of inadequate development time, a cool developer temperature, or a developer solution problem.

Overdeveloped Film

An overdeveloped film has a dark or high-density appearance (Fig. 7–34). It may be the result of excessive development time, an elevated developer temperature, or over-replenished or overconcentrated developer solution. For other possibilities and solutions, see the preceding paragraph.

Developer Solution Artifact

Dark spots are produced on the processed film when developer solution contacts the emulsion prior to film processing (Fig. 7–35). This type of artifact can be completely eliminated by maintaining a clean darkroom working surface, free of debris and chemical spills.

Fixer Solution Artifact

White spots are produced on the processed film when fixer solution contacts the emulsion prior to film processing (Fig. 7–36). This type of artifact can be

Figure 7–34. An overprocessed image has a dark, or high-density, appearance. It may be the result of excessive development time, an elevated developer temperature, or a developer solution problem.

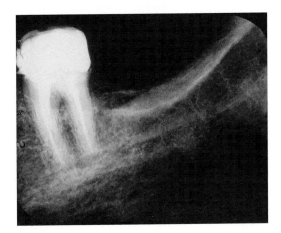

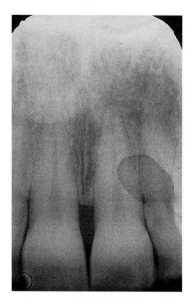

Figure 7-35. The dark spot on this film was caused by a droplet of developer solution that came in contact with the emulsion prior to film processing.

completely eliminated by maintaining a clean darkroom working surface, free of debris and chemical spills.

Yellow and Brown Stains

Yellow and brown stains on processed radiographs are usually the result of exhausted solutions, insufficient fixation, or inadequate washing. The most common stain is brown, which results from inadequate removal of the fixer solution from the emulsion (Fig. 7–37). The brown stain occurs over time as the remnant thiosulfate reacts with the metallic silver to form brown silver sulfide. These stains can be eliminated by washing the films for an adequate

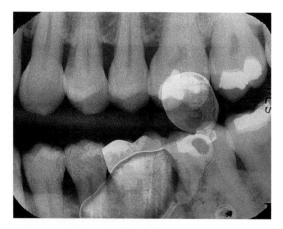

Figure 7-36. White artifacts are produced when fixer solution contacts the emulsion prior to film processing.

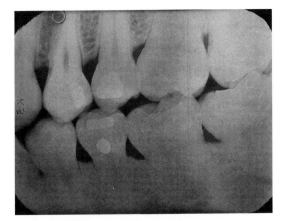

Figure 7–37. Brown stains are usually the result of inadequate washing of the film. The dark, mottled areas on this film would have a brown color in reflected light.

length of time in fresh, circulating water, ensuring adequate fixation, or replacing exhausted solutions with fresh chemicals.

Roller Marks

Marks and streaking of the emulsion may be caused by dirty rollers. Often these marks appear as dark vertical lines on the film emulsion (Fig. 7–38). Foreign debris, chemical deposits, or irregularities on the rollers are usually responsible for the artifacts. The rollers should be cleaned daily with a cleaning sheet and thoroughly cleaned each week and at every solution change. If the rollers have been abraded with abrasive cleaners and brushes,

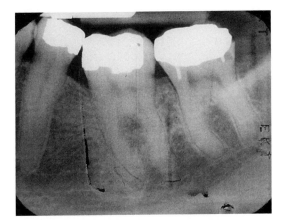

Figure 7–38. This film has a number of processing artifacts. The black vertical line between the second premolar and molar is a mark from another film contacting the emulsion; note the film edge configuration of the artifact. The dark vertical lines distal to each molar are artifacts from dirty rollers. Finally, a developer solution artifact is present near the roots of the second molar tooth.

they should be replaced, as the defects harbor debris and deposits that adversely affect the film.

REFERENCES

Bushong SC: Radiologic Science for Technologists: Physics, Biology, and Protection, 5th edition, pp 189–194. St. Louis, Mosby–Year Book, 1993.

Exposure and Processing for Dental Radiography. Rochester, New York, Eastman Kodak Company, 1994.

Goaz PW, White SC: Oral Radiology: Principles and Interpretation, 3rd edition, pp 106–125. St. Louis, Mosby–Year Book, 1994.

Haring JI, Lind LJ: Radiographic Interpretation for the Dental Hygienist, pp 159–180. Philadelphia, WB Saunders, 1993.

Langland OE, Langlais RP, Sippy FH, et al: Radiology for Dental Hygienists and Dental Assistants, pp 137–172. Springfield, Illinois, Charles C Thomas, 1988.

Management of Photographic Wastes in the Dental Office. Rochester, New York, Eastman Kodak Company, 1990.

Miles DA, Van Dis ML, Jensen CW, et al: Radiographic Imaging for Dental Auxiliaries, 2nd edition, pp 51–75. Philadelphia, WB Saunders, 1993.

Miles DA, Van Dis ML, Razmus TF: Basic Principles of Oral and Maxillofacial Radiology, pp 155–184. Philadelphia, WB Saunders, 1992.

Miller CH, Palenik CJ: Infection Control and Management of Hazardous Materials for the Dental Team, pp 230–247. St. Louis, Mosby–Year Book, 1994.

Quality Assurance in Dental Radiography. Rochester, New York, Eastman Kodak Company, 1995.

8

PANORAMIC RADIOGRAPHY, OTHER EXTRAORAL PROJECTIONS, AND IMPLANT SITE ASSESSMENT

THOMAS F. RAZMUS

Panoramic Imaging

Lateral Jaw Projections

Cephalometric Examinations

Paranasal Sinus Examinations

Temporomandibular Joint Examinations

Implant Site Assessment

This chapter presents a variety of ways to image large regions of the oral and maxillofacial complex, as well as limited, task-specific imaging techniques. The text briefly describes each technique along with its indications. Figures and legends present additional information about the application of the technique and assessment of image quality. Panoramic radiography has come to be the most widely used extraoral projection and is covered in more detail than the other extraoral projections. The section on implant site assessment, for the sake of completion, includes the application of intraoral techniques.

PANORAMIC IMAGING

Over the last half century, panoramic radiography has evolved into a valuable diagnostic tool for all health disciplines concerned with the oral and maxillofacial region. Extraction of accurate diagnostic information from panoramic images requires that the clinician first be capable of assessing the diagnostic quality of the panoramic radiograph at hand. Assessment of anatomic accuracy, a major element of diagnostic quality, requires an understanding of the relationship between the panoramic machine's image layer and how the patient is positioned in the machine. This section discusses the panoramic machine image layer, positioning the patient in the panoramic machine relative to its image layer, and the relationship between these elements and how they affect the anatomical accuracy and diagnostic quality of the resultant panoramic image. Image-degrading features resulting from errors in exposure or film processing may be described in certain figure legends but are not the main concern of this chapter.

The Image Layer and Positioning the Patient

Recall that panoramic radiography involves movement of the film and x-ray source (see Figure 1–2B) to produce a curved image plane of objects from

Table 8–1. Panoramic Patient Positioning and Associated Errors and Images

Positioning Element	Common Positioning Error Affecting the Element	Characteristic Image Appearance	Method of Error Correction
Midsagittal plane	Patient not centered in machine, head turned to one side, head canted to one side	Asymmetric width of molars and/or bicuspids from side-to-side, and/or image is diagonally oriented across film	Midsagittal plane (horizontal head position) centered in machine and perpendicular to the floor
Ala-tragus line (occlusal plane)	Chin too high or too low	Chin too high: flat occlusal plane, condyles near or off sides of film. Chin too low: excessive curve of occlusal plane, condyles near or off the top of the film	Ala-tragus line (vertical head position) positioned parallel to the floor
Anteroposterior (AP) position	Patient too far forward or too far back in the machine	Too far forward: anterior teeth blurred and narrower than expected. Too far back: anterior teeth blurred and wider than expected	Place midline between incisors into notch of bitepin or use whatever AP positioning aid is available on the machine being used
Cervical spine (neck) position	Neck angled or slumped forward	Radiopaque (white) shadow over images of anterior teeth, anterior teeth narrower than expected, spinal column visible on sides of image	Straighten cervical spine by having patient sit or stand erect

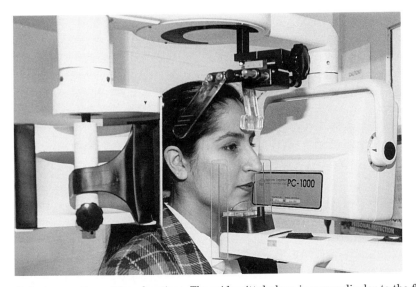

Figure 8–1. A correctly positioned patient. The midsagittal plane is perpendicular to the floor and centered between the acrylic lateral head positioners. The ala-tragus line (a horizontal line connecting the corner of the nose with the tab of the ear) is parallel to the floor. Anteroposterior positioning using manufacturer's guidelines will place the anterior teeth in the anterior segment of the image layer. The shoulders are relaxed and sloped downward. The cervical spine is erect. A space should exist between the shoulder and bottom edge of the cassette holder such that an open hand could be placed on the patient's shoulder under the cassette drum. All metallic objects above the neck should be removed. A lead apron designed for panoramic radiography should be placed over the patient's shoulders.

within the patient. The synchronized movement and relative speed of the film and x-ray source to each other result in a region in space, located between the film and x-ray source, called the *image layer.* The shape of the image layer of panoramic machines has been designed to correspond as closely as possible to the horseshoe shape of an average dental arch, including the condyles. When a patient is positioned in a panoramic machine in such a way that the dental arches and condyles are coincident with the machine's image layer, the sharpest and most anatomically accurate panoramic image of the patient will result. Positioning a patient so that the dental structures do not coincide with the image layer will generate images that exhibit anatomical distortions that are characteristic of the positioning error committed. In most cases, a patient positioned according to the machine manufacturer's instructions has dental arches and condyles located coincident with the image layer of the machine.

Table 8–1 lists the various elements of positioning a patient in a panoramic machine. Included are the significance of each positioning element, the most common error affecting each element, the characteristic appearance of the image produced by the error committed, and the method of eliminating the error from subsequent exposures.

Figures 8–1 through 8–10 illustrate various patient positioning situations in a typical panoramic machine. Images that are likely to result from each positioning scenario are presented. Technique errors other than those related to positioning a patient in the machine are described in the legend of the appropriate figures.

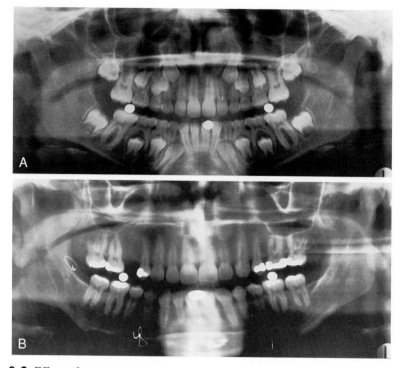

Figure 8–2. Effects of anteroposterior patient positioning on the resultant image. Radiopaque spherical objects placed at the center of the image layer will be imaged with minimal distortion and magnification. The anteriorly located ball bearing in *A* is relatively sharp and minimally distorted when compared with its counterpart in *B*. The anterior teeth in *A* are correspondingly sharper, less distorted, and less magnified than those in *B*. The skull in *A* was positioned according to the manufacturer's instructions relative to its anteroposterior location. The skull in *B* was positioned 3 mm back from the manufacturer's recommended location, and this resulted in unsharp and horizontally magnified images of the anterior teeth. The images of the ball bearings in the posterior regions remain spherical because no changes were introduced in lateral patient positioning. Additional features of a diagnostic quality panoramic image are given with Figure 8–4.

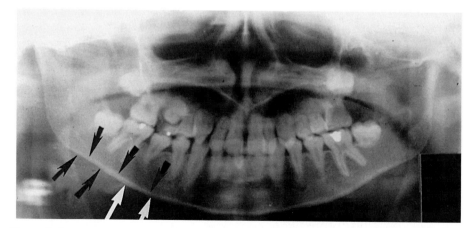

Figure 8–3. The "smile line," or gentle arc to the occlusal plane, indicates that the chin was correctly positioned in the superoinferior plane. Bilaterally symmetrical widths of premolar and molar crowns and rami indicate that the midsagittal plane was centered in the machine. Overlapping of the incisal edges of anterior teeth indicates that a bitepin or similar device was not used. The blurred and horizontally magnified images of the anterior teeth result from the patient being positioned farther back in the machine than recommended by the manufacturer, a situation similar to that in Figure 8–2*B*. The arrows delineate the mandibular inferior cortex.

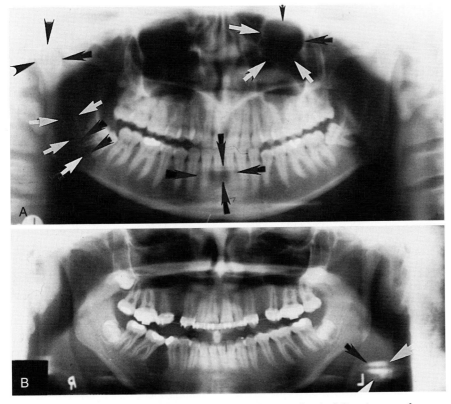

Figure 8–4. Images of a well-positioned patient. *A*, The arrowheads delineate several anatomical structures. At the upper left is the mandibular condyle. Progressing down the ramus, the mandibular or inferior alveolar canal is demonstrated. The arrows at the mandibular midline surround an artifact of the panoramic projection. Differentiation of such a radiolucency as an artifact or pathosis can be accomplished by making a periapical radiograph of the area. A panoramic projection artifact will not be present on the periapical radiograph. The arrows in the upper right surround the orbit.

B, The round radiopacity at the midline and between the incisal edges of the anterior teeth is the image of a plastic bitepin. Some panoramic machines are equipped with bitepins to aid in anteroposterior patient positioning. The arrows in the lower right corner point to the ghost image of the letter "R" from the opposite side of the radiograph.

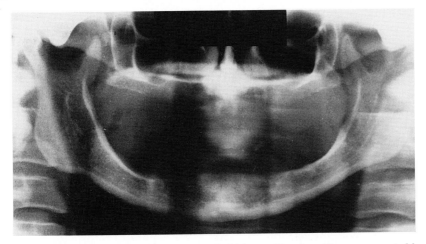

Figure 8–5. Image of an edentulous patient with fairly good head position as suggested by the gentle arc of the mandible. The bilateral images of the cervical spine indicate that the patient's neck was slumped or angled anteriorly, which placed the spine in the path of the beam. This patient, in all likelihood, was stretching forward to reach the bitepin or chinrest of the panoramic machine being used.

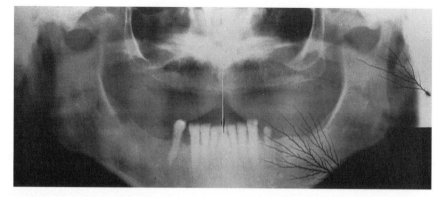

Figure 8–6. Image of a well-positioned, partially edentulous patient. The dark branching images resulted from static electricity, generated when the film was removed from its box or the cassette too rapidly.

LATERAL JAW PROJECTIONS

Lateral jaw radiographs are made to visualize either the body or the ramus of the mandible and are designated as the mandibular body and mandibular ramus views, respectively. The information provided by lateral jaw projections is available on panoramic radiographs, although the horizontal motion involved in making a panoramic image results in slightly less resolution than is provided by the static extraoral projection. A lateral jaw radiograph is an appropriate alternative when a panoramic machine is not accessible.

The mandibular body view demonstrates the teeth, alveolar bone, and inferior border of the mandible in the premolar-molar region. The ramus view is especially useful for assessment of the third molar region. This projection portrays the entire ramus by providing coverage up to and including the second mandibular molar, extending to below the mandibular angle, and superiorly to include the condyle. Figures 8–11 and 8–12 illustrate a patient positioned for each type of lateral jaw projection, along with a radiograph of each view.

CEPHALOMETRIC EXAMINATIONS

Cephalometric radiographs are made to demonstrate a side or a front view of the skull. These views are designated as a lateral or a posteroanterior (PA) view, respectively. Lateral and PA radiographs of the skull may be made that do not qualify for or fulfill the criteria of a cephalometric projection. Production of a cephalometric radiograph requires standardization of the way a patient is positioned in the cephalometric x-ray machine or apparatus. Lateral and PA cephalometric radiographs are made using a device called a *cephalostat*. This device helps position a patient in the machine the same way each time a new radiograph is made. The cephalostat provides a means to standardize, and thus to replicate, patient positioning from exposure to exposure.

The principal application of cephalometric radiography is in orthodontics, in which repetition of patient positioning is necessary to allow measurement of skeletal changes or growth and development over time. Cephalometric or noncephalometric lateral and PA skull views are also useful to assess (1) the sinuses, (2) the bones of the skull for signs of systemic disease or involvement by odontogenic or nonodontogenic lesions, and (3) potential implant sites. Figures 8–13 and 8–14 illustrate the lateral and PA skull techniques.

PARANASAL SINUS EXAMINATIONS

Evaluation of the sinuses in the skull using plain film radiography requires more than one view or projection. A panoramic radiograph often constitutes the initial exposure because it can provide broad coverage of the sinus anatomy, in particular the maxillary sinuses. A group of radiographic projections, sometimes designated as a *sinus series*, may be made to provide views in several imaging planes. A typical sinus series might include panoramic, Waters, posteroanterior (PA), submentovertex (SMV), and lateral skull radiographs. It is not uncommon for computed tomography (CT) or magnetic resonance (MR) imaging, or both, also to be employed.

Waters (Occipitomental) Projection

Although a panoramic radiograph is often the first image used to assess the maxillary sinuses, the Waters, or occipitomental, projection is considered to be the classic view for this application. In addition to the maxillary sinuses, the Waters view demonstrates the frontal and ethmoid sinuses, the orbit, the zygomaticofrontal suture, and the nasal cavity. Figure 8–15 illustrates a patient positioned for a Waters projection and a Waters radiographic image.

Posteroanterior (PA) Projection

This projection may be made with or without the use of a cephalostat. The PA view demonstrates the frontal and ethmoid sinuses, nasal fossae, and orbits. This view is useful to assess the skull for local or systemic disease involvement and to monitor growth and development. Serial measurements of growth and development should be assessed only from PA radiographs made using a cephalostat or other standardized criteria to assist in the replication of patient positioning from exposure to exposure. Figure 8–14 illustrates a patient positioned for a PA cephalometric projection and an example of the radiograph obtained. Although there is no obvious difference in a PA image made with or without a cephalostat, replication of patient positioning for serial exposures may not be reliable unless a cephalostat is employed.

Lateral Skull Projection

This view is useful to assess the skull and bones of the face for evidence of trauma, local or systemic disease involvement, or growth and development.

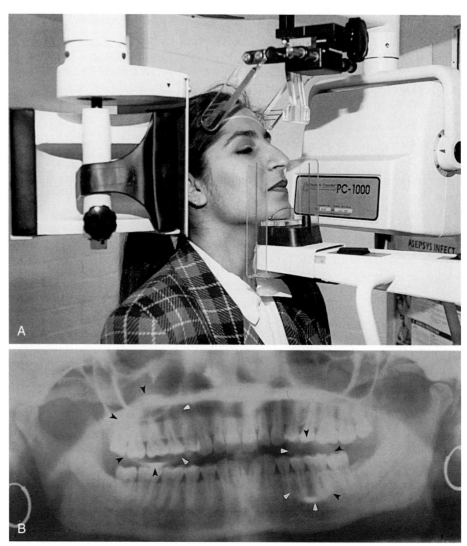

Figure 8–7. *A,* Patient positioned with the chin too high. Compare this position with that illustrated in Figure 8–1. Observe that when the chin is positioned too high, the maxillary anterior teeth will be moved upward, backward, and away from the center of the image layer. *B,* Image resulting when the chin is positioned too high. The occlusal plane becomes flattened and in extreme cases may exhibit a reversed curve of Spee. The condyles are projected toward the sides of the film and in extreme cases may be projected off the film. The radiopaque image of the hard palate may be projected over the roots of the maxillary teeth. An additional technique error was not having the patient remove the earrings. The real image of each earring appears at the side of the film. The ghost image (*arrows*) of each earring appears in the molar region on the side opposite its real image.

It can be made with or without a cephalostat. Repeated measurements from serial exposures are considered reliable only when standardized methods are used for positioning the patient. The most obvious difference between a lateral skull radiograph made according to cephalometric criteria and one made for general assessment is that the cephalometric image demonstrates the profile of the facial soft tissues. Figure 8–13 illustrates a lateral skull radiograph.

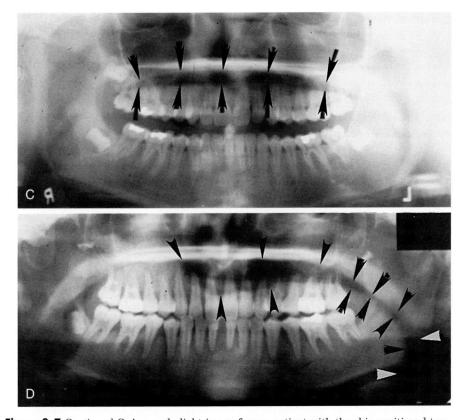

Figure 8–7 *Continued C*, An overly light image from a patient with the chin positioned too high. The result of an additional technique error is demonstrated by the dark area delineated by the arrows. Such an error results in loss of information about the root apices of the maxillary teeth and the floor of the maxillary sinus. This dark region represents the air space between the dorsum of the tongue and the hard palate, the palatoglossal air space. To prevent this error, patients must be carefully instructed to hold their entire tongue against the entire roof of their mouth while the machine is in motion. *D*, A situation similar to that in Figure 8–7C. This photo demonstrates a palatoglossal air space extending across part of the maxillary arch. Note the loss of information on the affected side. The arrowheads are delineating the air space between the soft palate and the dorsum of the tongue. The dark region traversing the ramus is called the oropharyngeal air space, a normal panoramic anatomical structure.

Submentovertex Projection

The SMV projection is also known as the basilar view. A submentovertex image demonstrates the base of the skull; the location, general shape, and orientation of the condyles; the sphenoid sinuses; the curvature of the dental arches and portions of the mandible; the lateral wall of the maxillary sinuses; and the zygomatic arches. Figure 8–16 illustrates a patient positioned for an SMV projection along with an example of an SMV image.

Additional Methods of Imaging the Paranasal Sinuses

Plain film tomography, computed tomography (CT), and magnetic resonance (MR) imaging are also used to assess the paranasal sinuses.

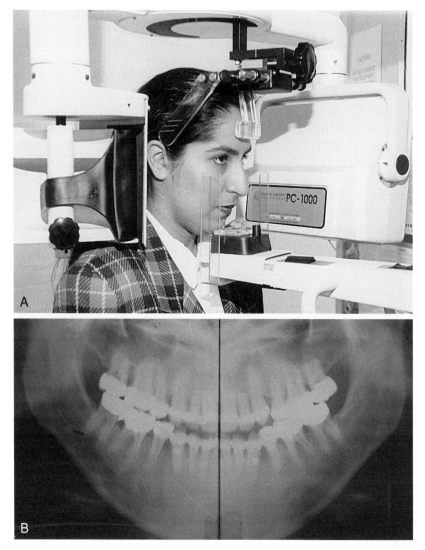

Figure 8–8. *A,* Patient positioned with the chin too low. Compare this with the position illustrated in Figure 8–1. The mandibular anterior teeth are moved backward, down, and away from the center of the image layer. *B,* Image from a patient positioned with the chin too low. The most obvious image characteristic of this positioning error is the increased curve of the occlusal plane and the projection of the condyles off the top of the film.

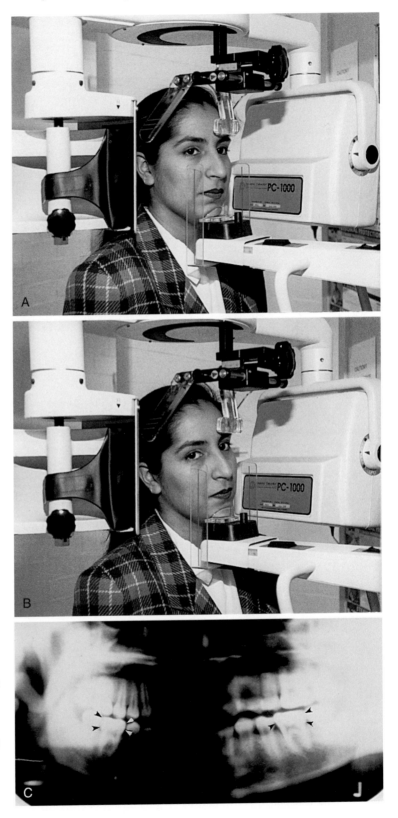

Figure 8-9. *A*, Patient positioned with the head turned to one side. *B*, Patient positioned with the head turned and canted to one side. *C*, Image resulting from the head being turned to one side. The ramus and teeth on the side to which the patient is turned will be too close to the film. The ramus and teeth on this side will be diminished in size (*left arrowheads*). The ramus and teeth on the opposite side will be too far away from the film and will be magnified (*right arrowheads*). Such an image is completely distorted.

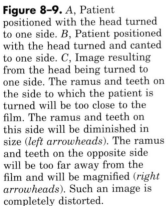

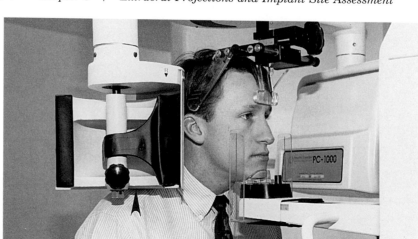

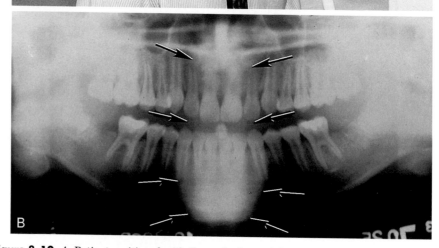

Figure 8–10. *A,* Patient positioned with the neck slumped forward. The film cassette carrier is also in contact with the patient's shoulder (*arrow*), which may hinder movement of the machine. *B,* A slumped-neck position will result in the cervical spine being imaged as the oblong, vertical radiopacity in the middle of the image, as delineated by the arrows. In extreme cases the anatomical structures in this area of the radiograph can be completely obliterated.

Tomography employing intensifying screens and light-sensitive film systems is most useful for the evaluation of bone associated with suspected sinus pathosis. Disruption or distortion of the walls and floor of the sinuses can be well visualized. Soft tissue anatomy and lesions within the sinus cavity may be detectable as a subtle change in radiodensity.

Computed tomography, as does plain film tomography, employs x rays to create an image. The computerized image acquisition and manipulation capabilities of CT allow much more information to be collected, processed, and presented for evaluation than plain film tomography. CT has the capability to image soft tissue and subtle qualitative changes of bone. CT is useful for assessing the extent of disease in chronic or recurrent sinusitis patients. The

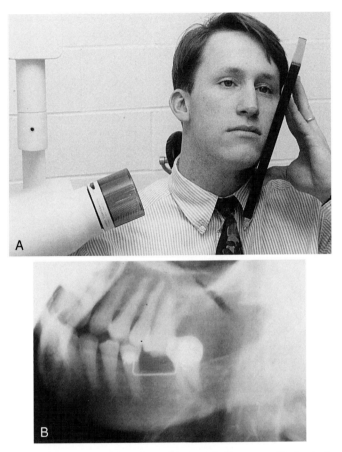

Figure 8-11. *A*, Patient positioned for a lateral jaw projection—mandibular body view. Note that the film cassette is against the body of the mandible. *B*, Lateral jaw radiograph of the mandibular body.

data in the CT computer can be used to create three-dimensional images of sinus anatomy and associated abnormalities in preparation for surgery.

Magnetic resonance imaging is the best modality to apply for visualization and differentiation of adjacent soft tissue masses. The mechanism of MR imaging provides data that are associated with the chemical make-up of the structures being imaged. Such data allow the demonstration of neoplasms infiltrating into adjacent or surrounding soft tissues, as well as information about the composition of the lesion.

TEMPOROMANDIBULAR JOINT EXAMINATIONS

Several plain film techniques are useful to image the temporomandibular joint (TMJ). Computed tomography and magnetic resonance imaging provide additional diagnostic information as well as added capacity for image enhancement through computer manipulation of image data.

The standard panoramic radiograph can provide a *noncorrected* tomo-

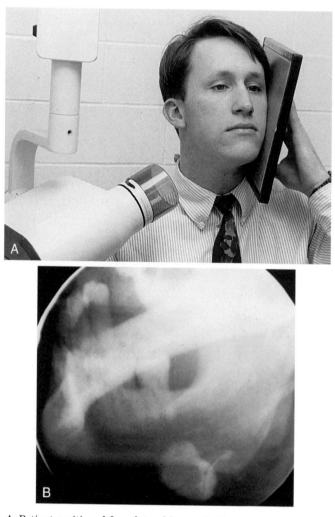

Figure 8-12. *A,* Patient positioned for a lateral jaw projection—ramus view. Note that the film cassette is against the ramus. *B,* Lateral jaw radiograph of the ramus.

graphic view of both condyles on one film. The condylar image is designated as noncorrected because the x-ray beam does not pass through the long axis of the condyle. The long axis of the average condyle is oriented at approximately 20° to the coronal plane, with the medial pole angled posteriorly. This orientation results in distortion of the condylar image in panoramic projections. Panoramic images should be reserved for assessment of gross osseous changes of the condyle. Several panoramic machines are capable of exposing specialized TMJ views that portray up to four images on one film; open and closed views can be made of each condyle. These projections require that the patient's normal panoramic head position be altered: the head is moved slightly forward and turned toward the side of interest. This maneuver positions the long axis of the condyle of interest approximately parallel to the path of the x-ray beam. A panoramic TMJ radiograph is illustrated in Figure 8–17.

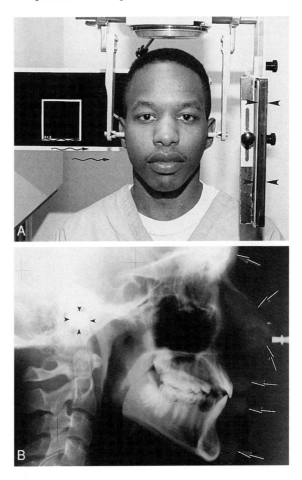

Figure 8–13. *A,* Patient positioned for a lateral cephalometric radiograph. The film cassette is to the patient's left (*large arrowheads*). The x-ray source (*wavy arrows*) is to the patient's right. The ear rods (*small arrowheads*) of the cephalostat help reproduce patient positioning for serial radiographs. *B,* Lateral cephalometric radiograph. Note the facial soft tissue profile (*arrows*) and the superimposed ear rod images (*small arrowheads*).

Transcranial Projection

Clinicians often differ in their opinion of the utility of this view for assessing the TMJ. The image produced is especially subject to geometric distortion arising from variations in the patient's head position and in the vertical and horizontal angulation of the x-ray beam. Devices exist to aid in replicating the patient's head position between serial exposures. Use of such an apparatus can contribute a degree of consistency when obtaining serial images. The transcranial view can be used to evaluate the cortical outline of the superior surface of the condyle and the cortical outline of the eminence, to visualize the degree of translation of the condyle, and to make a general statement about the joint space. Plain film lateral tomography is rapidly replacing transcranial radiography. Figure 8–18 presents an example of transcranial radiography.

Transpharyngeal Projection

The transpharyngeal view has indications and limitations similar to those of the transcranial projection. Its principal use is to visualize the cortical outline of the condyle from its lateral aspect. Figure 8–19 illustrates a transpharyngeal radiograph.

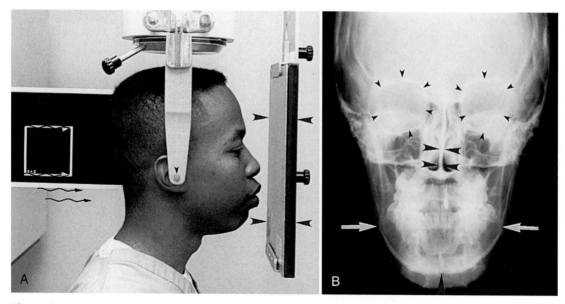

Figure 8-14. *A,* Patient positioned for a posteroanterior (PA) cephalometric radiograph. The patient is facing the film cassette (*large arrowheads*). The x-ray source (*wavy arrows*) is behind the patient. The cephalostat and its ear rods (*small arrowhead*) facilitate reproducible patient positioning. *B,* A posteroanterior (PA) cephalometric radiograph. Facial skeletal structures are imaged the sharpest because they are positioned closest to the film. Orbits are outlined by small arrowheads. Nasal septum is between four large arrowheads. Gonial angles are indicated by arrows. Chinpoint is marked.

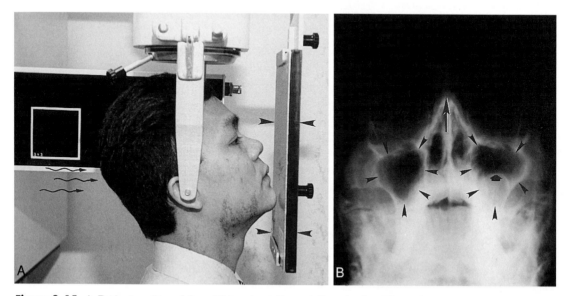

Figure 8-15. *A,* Patient positioned for a Waters (occipitomental) projection. The patient is facing the film cassette (*large arrowheads*), the nose is approximately 2 inches from the cassette, and the chin is nearly in contact with the cassette. The x-ray source (*wavy arrows*) is behind the patient. *B,* Waters radiographic image. Maxillary sinuses are outlined by small arrowheads. The tip of the nose is indicated by the black and white arrow. A dome-shaped radiopacity occupying the lower half of the maxillary sinus is indicated by the fat arrow.

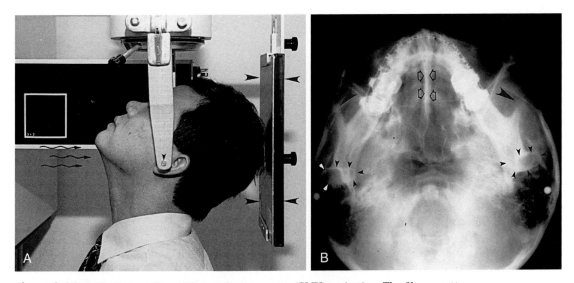

Figure 8-16. *A,* Patient positioned for a submentovertex (SMV) projection. The film cassette (*large arrowheads*) is behind the patient. The patient's neck is extended as far as practical to allow the x-ray beam (*wavy arrows*) to pass as closely perpendicular as possible to the superimposed dental arches. The cephalostat and ear rods (*small arrowhead*) are not necessary but help position the patient symmetrically in the machine. This is especially significant when the resultant SMV image is to be used in conjunction with tomography. *B,* SMV (basilar) radiograph. The bilateral radiopaque spheres mark the location of the ear rods in the external ear canals. Condyles are outlined by small arrowheads. Coronoid processes are indicated by large arrowheads. The midpalatal suture is between four open arrows.

Transorbital Projection

When frontal tomography is not available, the transorbital radiograph is the frontal projection of choice to visualize the structures comprising the condylar complex. Transorbital as well as transcranial and transpharyngeal radiographs are often made with the mouth open and closed. Transcranial and transpharyngeal radiographs made with the patient's mouth open can provide information about the degree of condylar translation and can demonstrate anatomical information about the condyle and eminence not available on a closed-mouth image.

An open mouth transorbital projection allows visualization of the articulating surface of the eminence and the condyle from its medial to lateral pole. A closed-mouth view results in these structures being at least partially superimposed on each other and obscured. The condylar neck can be evaluated on either an open or closed-mouth transorbital view. The open mouth transorbital technique demonstrates the most anatomy and is the view of choice. Figure 8–20 illustrates a transorbital radiograph.

Plain Film Tomography

Tomography is the plain film radiographic technique that provides the most definitive diagnostic information about the osseous components of the TMJ. Tomographic images may be made as lateral or frontal views.

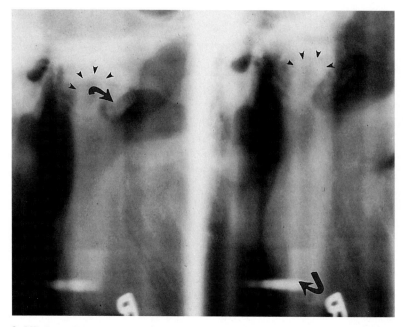

Figure 8–17. Specialized panoramic temporomandibular joint (TMJ) projections. The image on the left was made with the mouth closed, and the image on the right with the mouth open. The condyle has moved down and forward in the open mouth view. The direction of condylar movement is indicated by the curved arrow in the left image. The direction of gonial angle movement is indicated by the curved arrow in the right image. The superior aspect of the condyle in each view is outlined by arrowheads.

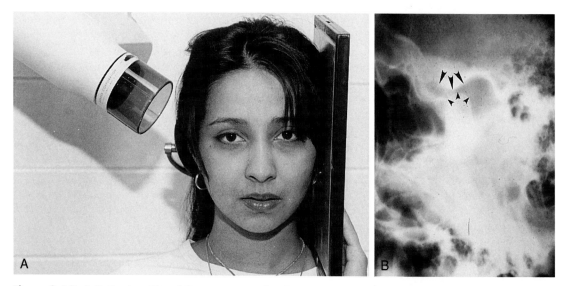

Figure 8–18. *A,* Patient positioned for a transcranial radiograph of the left side condyle. *B,* Transcranial radiographic image: open mouth view. The articular eminence is delineated by large arrowheads. The condyle is delineated by small arrowheads.

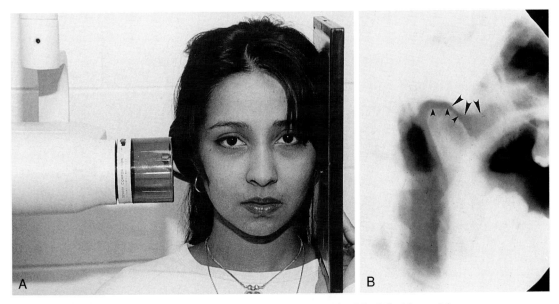

Figure 8–19. *A,* Patient positioned for a transpharyngeal radiograph of the left side condyle. *B,* Transpharyngeal radiographic image: closed mouth view. The articular eminence is delineated by large arrowheads. The condyle is delineated by small arrowheads.

Lateral and frontal tomographic views are commonly corrected for the angulation of the condyles by applying a few simple measurements and calculations to an SMV image of the patient. Resultant data can then be applied to adjust the position of the patient in the tomographic machine so that the central ray of the x-ray beam will be aligned to pass parallel to and through the long axis of the condyle. Rather than calculate the precise angulation of the condyles from an SMV image, the patient's head can be rotated 20° to 25° toward the side of interest. Such a maneuver is often adequate to produce an approximate corrected lateral view of the condyle. This technique provides a relatively simple means of obtaining a scout tomographic film of a condyle.

Lateral tomograms are useful to visualize the anterior, superior, and posterior cortical outline of the condyles, the cortical outline of the mandibular fossa and eminence, and the degree of condylar translation. Frontal tomograms allow clear visualization of the superior surface of the condylar head. Both lateral and frontal tomograms can demonstrate the subtle cortical changes associated with arthritis. Figure 8–21 is an example of tomographic TMJ images.

Computed Tomography

Computed tomography excels at imaging the osseous structures of the TMJ. It can generate superior images of the head of the condyle, the articular eminence, and the mandibular fossa. The ability to reconstruct CT data into three-dimensional images makes the modality especially useful in the analysis of fractures of the condylar head and neck. Computed tomography has

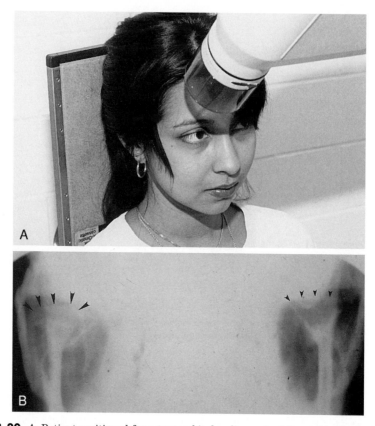

Figure 8–20. *A,* Patient positioned for a transorbital radiograph of the right side condyle. *B,* Transorbital radiographic image. This bilateral open mouth view demonstrates the superior surface of the condyle on the left side of the image (*large arrowheads*), but the condyle on the opposite side (*small arrowheads*) remains partially hidden. This finding suggests that only the condyle on the left side of the image has undergone translation upon opening. A bilateral technique such as this precludes the making of images corrected for condylar angulation.

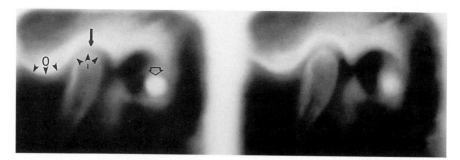

Figure 8–21. Plain film tomographic TMJ images. The open arrow indicates the metal ball at the end of the ear rod. The difference in sharpness of the ball between images indicates that each image was made at a different depth of cut. Arrowheads at "0" delineate the articular eminence. Arrowheads at "1" delineate the condyle. The solid black arrow indicates the roof of the glenoid fossa. (Courtesy of Dr. Robert G. Pifer, West Virginia University School of Dentistry, Morgantown, West Virginia.)

largely been replaced by magnetic resonance imaging for visualizing the soft tissues in the joint. Figure 8–22 is an example of a CT image of a temporomandibular joint.

Magnetic Resonance Imaging

Magnetic resonance imaging can produce high-quality images of the articular disk and its attachments, the muscles, the condyle, and the mandibular fossa in the same image. Variation of technique parameters can be applied to visualize inflammatory joint changes, joint effusion, disk position, disk shape, bone changes, hard and soft tissue changes associated with joint implants, as well as the joint in motion. Figure 8–23 is an example of a magnetic resonance TMJ image.

IMPLANT SITE ASSESSMENT

Imaging modalities useful in implant dentistry include panoramic radiography, plain film tomography, computed tomography, and film-based periapical and intraoral direct digital radiography. Different views and techniques are necessary to assess adequately the height, width, and configuration of the bone associated with the proposed site. A presurgical imaging assessment is

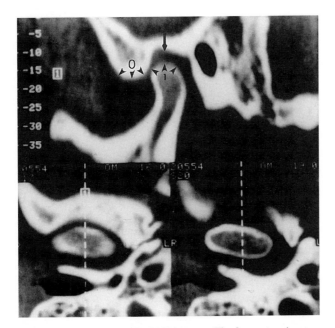

Figure 8–22. Computed tomographic (CT) TMJ images. The lower two images are axial projections made of the patient. The lateral view in the top half of the photograph was reconstructed from axial image data by computer manipulation and multiplanar reformatting. Arrowheads at "0" delineate the articular eminence. Arrowheads at "1" delineate the condyle. The black arrow indicates the roof of the glenoid fossa. (Courtesy of Dr. S. Brent Dove, University of Texas Dental School at San Antonio, Texas.)

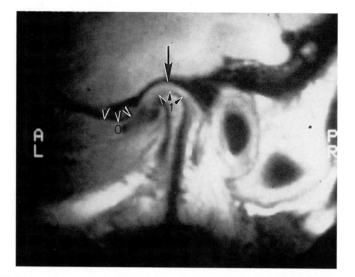

Figure 8–23. Magnetic resonance (MR) TMJ image. MR does not depend on x-ray attenuation to produce images. MR images demonstrate structures relative to their hydrogen ion (water) content. Bone contains very little water and is imaged as a dark region on MR images. Soft tissues contain varying amounts of water and will exhibit proportionally bright images. Arrowheads at "0" indicate the articular eminence or tubercle; the dark region is the temporal bone. Arrowheads at "1" indicate the cortex of the condyle. The gray area within the dark cortical signal is bone marrow, which exhibits a significant water content. The large arrow indicates the roof of the glenoid fossa of the temporal bone. Compare this image with those produced using x rays. (Courtesy of Dr. S. Brent Dove, University of Texas Dental School at San Antonio, Texas.)

concerned with the quantity and quality of bone and the location of critical anatomical structures. Postsurgical images are useful to help determine the optimal time for the second stage procedure. Postsurgical, postloading, and follow-up imaging address the status of integration or "bone fill" around the implant. Follow-up assessment helps monitor bone height and configuration and the status of the bone-implant interface.

Intraoral Imaging

Film-based periapical and occlusal radiographs, as well as direct digital radiography, provide the best image detail and sharpest images, minimal geometrical distortion, and the least magnification if the operator diligently applies the principles of the intraoral paralleling technique. Intraoral imaging can provide information about bone quality, such as density and trabecular pattern. Measurements of bone height, and the distance between and from critical anatomical structures, can be considered accurate when made on an image that resulted from precise image receptor placement.

Disadvantages of intraoral imaging include a high potential for operator-induced image distortion, which will affect the accuracy of measurements and the reproducibility of serial radiographs used to monitor treatment outcomes. Intraoral images can provide information about the mesiodistal and superoinferior dimensions only, leaving the buccolingual dimension unexplored.

Figure 8–24 portrays the bone-implant interface in direct digital image format.

Panoramic Radiography

Panoramic radiography can provide information about bone quality, such as density and trabecular pattern, at multiple implant sites. Findings that are local or remote to the site(s), such as odontogenic or nonodontogenic lesions, manifestations of systemic disease, condylar changes, and so on that may compromise treatment outcomes, can be assessed.

A concern with panoramic radiography, as with all forms of imaging, is accurate positioning of the patient in the machine. Panoramic images, in particular, often exhibit distortions resulting from errors in patient positioning. The clinician must be able to recognize when these image distortions are present, know the associated error, and know how to eliminate the error from a subsequent exposure. Unless the clinician is competent in assessing the diagnostic quality of a panoramic image in this way, information obtained from the image may be inaccurate. Earlier in this chapter and in Chapter 1 additional information about the assessment of the diagnostic quality of panoramic images was presented.

A panoramic image of a well-positioned patient exhibits certain features inherent in the technique. Magnification and a lack of sharpness will always be present to some degree. The exact magnification factor is provided in the owner's manual accompanying the machine and may range from 10% to 30%.

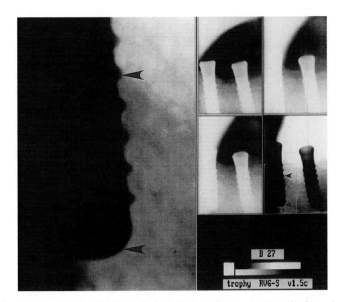

Figure 8–24. Computer-assisted (direct digital) images demonstrating the bone-implant interface. The large arrowheads in the enlarged image correspond to the small arrowheads within the "window" of the original projection at the lower right hand corner. Note that the images referred to are displayed with their contrast (black and white areas) reversed; the remaining images exhibit conventional contrast. (Courtesy of Dr. T. Parks, Indiana University School of Dentistry, Indianapolis.)

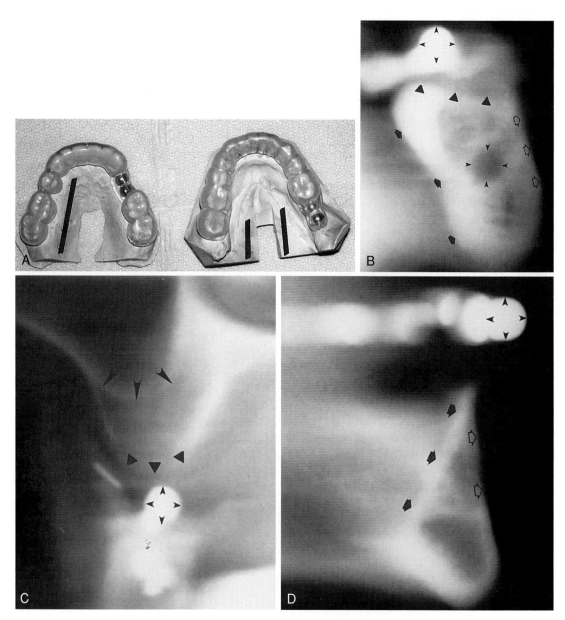

Figure 8–25. *A,* Two examples of acrylic stents that will place a spherical metallic indicator over the proposed implant site(s). Stents with metal indicators cannot be used for CT imaging because of the production of scatter artifact in the image. (Courtesy of Dr. T. Parks, Indiana University School of Dentistry, Indianapolis.) *B,* Spherical image of a metal ball to confirm slice location at a proposed mandibular posterior implant site. The image of a metal ball is delineated by small arrowheads. The alveolar ridge crest is delineated by triangles. Lingual cortical bone is marked by solid fat arrows. Buccal cortical bone is delineated by open arrows. The mandibular (inferior alveolar nerve) canal is outlined by small arrowheads. (Courtesy of Dr. J. Katz, University of Missouri at Kansas City School of Dentistry, Kansas City, Missouri.) *C,* Spherical image of a metal ball to confirm slice location at a proposed maxillary posterior implant site. The floor of the maxillary sinus is delineated by large arrowheads. The alveolar ridge crest is outlined by triangles. The image of a metal ball is delineated by small arrowheads. (Courtesy of Dr. J. Katz, University of Missouri at Kansas City School of Dentistry, Kansas City, Missouri.) *D,* Spherical image of a metal ball to confirm slice location at a proposed mandibular anterior implant site. Note that this image also confirms a knife-edge configuration of the anterior edentulous ridge. The image of a metal ball is delineated by small arrowheads. Lingual cortical bone is delineated by solid arrows. Buccal cortical bone is delineated by open arrows. (Courtesy of Dr. J. Katz, University of Missouri at Kansas City School of Dentistry, Kansas City, Missouri.)

Lack of sharpness is a feature of tomography, which results from the motion of the film and x-ray source. In panoramic radiography, the motion is limited to the horizontal plane around the patient. Horizontal measurements should not be made on panoramic radiographs. The vertical x-ray beam angulation of panoramic machines is fixed, and the projection geometry in the vertical plane is analogous to that of intraoral radiography. Vertical measurements on panoramic images can be considered accurate. As with intraoral imaging, no information is provided about the buccolingual dimension.

Plain Film Tomography

Conventional tomography has come to be the most cost-effective imaging technique for implant site assessment. It provides the greatest information yield, is area-specific and task-oriented, allows precise and reproducible measurements incorporating a constant magnification factor, and provides visualization of the buccolingual dimension. The technique produces a "slice" of information from a preselected image layer within the patient that can be 2.0 mm or more in thickness. Structures of interest in the image layer are better visualized due to increased contrast and resolution.

An acrylic stent with radiopaque indicators, such as ball-bearings, threaded screws, gutta-percha, or wire shapes placed above potential implant sites, is helpful when evaluating the tomogram. A sharp and nondistorted image of the radiopaque object confirms that the image being observed was made at the intended location. Figure 8–25 provides an example of an acrylic stent and images illustrating the use of radiopaque indicators to confirm the location of the image slice.

Disadvantages of conventional tomography may include limited access to a machine and the need for an oral and maxillofacial radiologist to interpret the resultant images.

The film-based imaging modalities discussed in this section represent the state-of-the-art in imaging technology, but none of these techniques provides for the easy visualization of subtle or early changes of bone adjacent to the implant. Computer-assisted subtraction radiography has been applied to the quantification of bone status at the implant interface.

Computed Tomography

The general principles of CT were discussed in Chapter 1. When a CT examination is to be made for implant site assessment, the patient is put into the CT unit in a supine position. The arch to be imaged must be positioned perpendicular to the floor, and the patient's head must be restrained to maintain this position throughout the scan. The axial images obtained are than subjected to computer manipulation via multiplanar reformatting to generate cross-sectional and panoramic images. Additional computer manipulations can create three-dimensional images from the two-dimensional image data that were collected from the patient. Figures 1–13 and 8–26 and 8–27 illustrate examples of CT imaging for implant site assessment. Table 8–2 presents a suggested imaging protocol for implant dentistry.

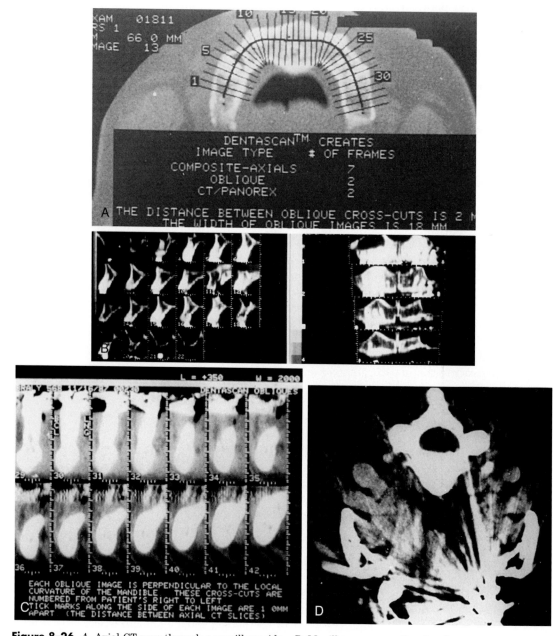

Figure 8–26. *A,* Axial CT scan through a maxillary ridge. *B,* Maxillary cross-sectional and panoramic images reconstructed from the axial image in *A. C,* Mandibular cross-sectional images reconstructed from an axial image similar to Figure 1–13*A. D,* Scatter artifact that occurs when a CT image is made in the proximity of metallic objects, such as restorations or metallic indicators in a stent. (Courtesy of Dr. S. Brent Dove, University of Texas Dental School at San Antonio, Texas.)

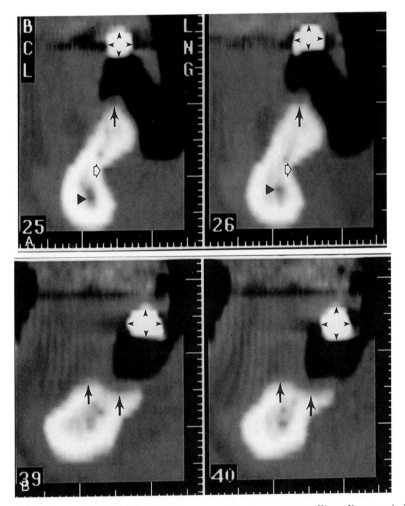

Figure 8–27. CT presurgical implant site assessment using a nonmetallic radiopaque indicator (*small arrowheads*) to confirm image slice location. Numbers in the lower left corner correspond to the slice location from axial image CT data. Buccal (BCL) and lingual (LNG) bone surfaces are indicated. Alveolar crest bone is indicated by large arrows in both *A* and *B*. In *A*, a lingual concavity is indicated by an open arrow and a critical anatomical structure (inferior alveolar nerve canal) by the triangular arrow. (Courtesy of Dr. T. Parks, Indiana University School of Dentistry, Indianapolis.)

Table 8–2. Suggested Imaging for Implant Dentistry

Presurgical Assessment	Postplacement, Postloading, and Periodic Monitoring
Periapical radiography	Periapical radiography
Panoramic radiography	Panoramic radiography
Plain film tomography	Plain film tomography
Direct digital imaging	Direct digital imaging
Computed tomography using nonmetallic indicators if no metallic restorations are in the proximity	

REFERENCES

Brooks SL: Computed tomography. Dent Clin North Am 1993;37(4):575–590.

Bushong SC: Special x-ray equipment and procedures. In Radiologic Science for Technologists: Physics, Biology, and Protection, 4th edition, p 308. St. Louis, CV Mosby, 1988.

Bushong SC: Computed tomography. In Radiologic Science for Technologists: Physics, Biology, and Protection, 4th edition, p 385. St. Louis, CV Mosby, 1988.

Bushong SC: Physical principles of magnetic resonance imaging. In Radiologic Science for Technologists: Physics, Biology, and Protection, 4th edition, p 409. St. Louis, CV Mosby, 1988.

Bushong SC: Magnetic resonance equipment and images. In Radiologic Science for Technologists: Physics, Biology, and Protection, 4th edition, p 427. St. Louis, CV Mosby, 1988.

Dove SB, McDavid WD: Digital panoramic and extraoral imaging. Dent Clin North Am 1993;37(4):541–551.

Edwards MK: Magnetic resonance imaging of the head and neck. Dent Clin North Am 1993;37(4):591–611.

Farman AG, Nortjé CJ, Wood RE: Principles of image interpretation. In Goaz PW, White SC: Oral Radiology: Principles and Interpretation, 3rd edition, p 291. St. Louis, CV Mosby, 1994.

Frederiksen NL: Specialized radiographic techniques. In Goaz PW, White SC: Oral Radiology: Principles and Interpretation, 3rd edition, p 266. St. Louis, CV Mosby, 1994.

Goaz PW, White SC: Extraoral radiographic examinations. In Oral Radiology: Principles and Interpretation, 3rd edition, p 227. St. Louis, CV Mosby, 1994.

Gratt BM: Panoramic radiography. In Goaz PW, White SC: Oral Radiology: Principles and Interpretation, 3rd edition, p 242. St. Louis, CV Mosby, 1994.

Gratt BM, Shetty V: Implant radiology. In Goaz PW, White SC: Oral Radiology: Principles and Interpretation, 3rd edition, p 703. St. Louis, CV Mosby, 1994.

Kassebaum DK, Nummikoski PV, Triplett RG, et al: Cross-sectional radiography for implant site assessment. Oral Surg Oral Med Oral Pathol 1990;70(5):674–678.

Miles DA: Plain film extraoral radiographic techniques. In Miles DA, Van Dis ML, Razmus TF: Basic Principles of Oral and Maxillofacial Radiology, p 123. Philadelphia, WB Saunders, 1992.

Razmus TF: Advanced imaging modalities. In Miles DA, Van Dis ML, Razmus TF: Basic Principles of Oral and Maxillofacial Radiology, p 185. Philadelphia, WB Saunders, 1992.

Razmus TF, Glass BJ, McDavid WD: Comparison of image layer location among panoramic machines of the same manufacturer. Oral Surg Oral Med Oral Pathol 1989;67:102–108.

Schwarz MS, Rothman SLG, Chafetz N, et al: Computed tomography in dental implantation surgery. Dent Clin North Am 1989;33(4):555–597.

9

RADIOGRAPHIC INTERPRETATION—DESCRIBING WHAT YOU SEE

T H O M A S   F.   R A Z M U S

Viewing Conditions

Descriptive Terminology

Radiographic Assessment

Radiographic and other forms of diagnostic image findings must be correlated with past and present patient data for the diagnostic process to be effective. Sources of past and present patient information include the medical and dental histories, clinical examination, existing diagnostic images, clinical laboratory tests, and the chief complaint. The correlation process requires that the clinician possess a knowledge base that will allow relationships among data from various sources to be recognized. The ability to correlate radiographic data with other information and to express the results in a meaningful and consistent fashion requires a level of communication skill in radiographic description. Chapter 9 has been designed to provide the novice clinician with a limited amount of experience in the communication of radiographic findings. The discussion will introduce (1) the essentials of optimal radiographic viewing conditions, (2) some very basic but standardized terminology to help the novice develop a consistent method of describing what appears on a radiograph, and (3) several radiographic images along with a description of the radiographic findings.

VIEWING CONDITIONS

The practice of dentistry often involves the observation of subtle and extremely small structural changes or variations from normal. A well-performed intraoral examination provides access to only a portion of the data available about the teeth and surrounding bone; the radiographic examination will provide a major portion of the remaining data. A clinician would not consider an intraoral clinical examination to be accurate or complete if it were performed without the proper light source and instrumentation. The same principle applies to a radiographic examination. The maximum amount of information contained in a radiographic examination is not likely to be appreciated by the observer if the images are not viewed under the correct conditions.

Information yield from radiographs placed on a viewbox in a busy and brightly lit operatory will be compromised, and small, subtle findings are more likely to be overlooked, especially if the images were not previously studied under appropriate conditions. Radiographs held up to lights in the ceiling are even less likely to yield complete information. Radiographs to be utilized at chairside during patient treatment should be studied under the appropriate viewing conditions and reviewed shortly before beginning treatment for the day.

A few simple practices, which should become habitual, will help the clinician obtain the maximum amount of information from radiographic examinations. Radiographic information obtained under the following environmental conditions, coupled with a clinical examination and history, is most likely to provide the operator with a comprehensive patient assessment.

1. **Viewing room**: Background lighting should be dim; the observer should allow the eyes to adjust to the darkened environment before reading the radiographs.

2. **Viewbox**: Should be of adequate size to accommodate the largest film used in the office; brightness should be uniform across the entire viewing surface.

3. **Opaque viewbox mask**: Used to block extraneous light from around a radiograph when the film size does not cover the entire viewing surface of the viewbox. A mask can be made from a piece of cardboard or an exposed and processed film large enough to cover the surface of the viewbox. A hole is cut in the mask the size of the film to be read, allowing light to pass only through the radiographs. It may be necessary to have different masks available to accommodate a mounted full mouth survey, a panoramic radiograph, or a periapical radiograph, and so on.

4. **Hot-light**: A special-purpose, high-intensity lamp with a continuously variable brightness control; used to examine overly dense areas of a radiographic image.

DESCRIPTIVE TERMINOLOGY

A clinician providing a diagnostic radiology service should be able to provide a concise and consistent description of any given radiographic presentation. The description should be such that another clinician would be able to formulate a relatively accurate mental picture of the situation at hand. Although the key terms used in a radiographic description should represent diagnostically significant information, the ability to generate a radiographic description does not require the expertise to arrive at a diagnosis.

Mastery of a fairly limited list of terms will allow the practitioner to formulate concise and consistent descriptions of almost any radiographic presentation. A scheme for generating a radiographic description is suggested here. For a telephone consultation that will involve a discussion of radiographic findings, a written description should be recorded beforehand.

The following elements should be stated:

- The type of projection:
  periapical radiograph
  panoramic radiograph, and so on

- The location:
  focal (isolated) or single
    associated with teeth: pericoronal, periapical
    in bone and not associated with teeth
  multifocal or in several locations
  generalized alteration of bone

- The external shape and internal architecture:
  unilocular (round or ovoid)
  multilocular (scalloped or lobulated)
  irregular

- The general radiographic features:
  radiolucent (dark)
  radiopaque (light)
  mixed radiolucent/radiopaque (dark and light within the same lesion)

- The character of the borders:
  sharply outlined: corticated, noncorticated
  indistinct or ragged

- The size (greatest dimensions):
  small (<1.0 cm)
  large (>1.0 cm)

- Alteration of adjacent structures:
  distortion by
    cortical expansion
    displacement of teeth
  destruction by
    cortical perforation
    resorption of teeth

Stating the type of projection can help the report recipient visualize the image format. A focal (single) lesion will have different ramifications than multifocal lesions (those that occur at multiple sites). A lesion associated with a tooth or teeth raises a significantly different list of questions for the diagnostician than a lesion located in bone and isolated from the teeth. A round or ovoid lesion, in many cases, will not exhibit internal compartments or septa, whereas one with a scalloped or lobulated shape is likely to have some sort of internal architecture. A generalized alteration of bone raises the possibility of systemic involvement.

The x-ray attenuation properties of the area of interest determine the degree of radiopacity or radiolucency exhibited by the image. A radiolucent lesion containing calcified material exhibits areas of radiopacity within the radiolucency and thus is described as a mixed radiolucent/radiopaque lesion. A sharply delineated lesion with a corticated outline has a border that appears white or radiopaque. An area that is sharply delineated but noncorticated exhibits a well-defined transition from the adjacent area but not a white outline.

When an indistinct or ragged outline comprises the borders of a lesion, it is difficult to differentiate exactly where the lesion begins and ends. The size of the lesion is determined using a millimeter ruler. Width and height are measured and recorded in millimeters or centimeters.

An abnormal development within the bones of the oral and maxillofacial complex takes on special significance when distortion or destruction of adjacent structures is demonstrated on the radiographs. Lesions that appear to be moving teeth or causing resorption of tooth roots are relatively easy to recognize. Determination of cortical expansion requires proficiency in radiographic anatomy and is beyond the capabilities of most novice radiographers.

RADIOGRAPHIC ASSESSMENT

This section consists of radiographic images and accompanying legends that apply the basic elements of a radiographic description. If the reader finds that the anatomical terminology used in this section is unfamiliar, an atlas of dental radiographic anatomy or similar reference should be consulted.

Text continued on page 279

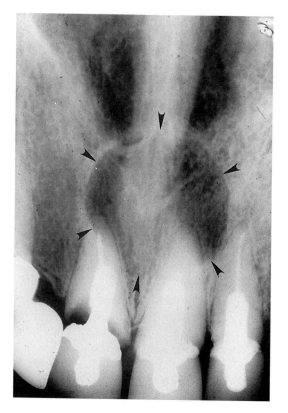

Figure 9–1. A periapical radiograph of the maxillary midline, demonstrating a single, round, unilocular radiolucency *(arrowheads)*, with a corticated outline and associated with the root apices of teeth numbers 8 and 9. The radiolucent area inside the borders appears to be occupied by a continuation of the adjacent normal bone trabecular pattern. The lesion is approximately 1.0 cm in diameter. The lamina dura and periodontal ligament (PDL) space do not appear to be affected.

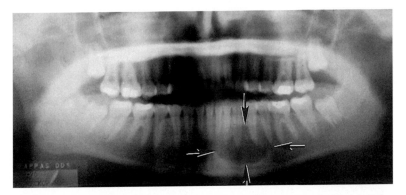

Figure 9–2. A panoramic radiograph demonstrating a single, ovoid, unilocular radiolucency *(arrows)*, with continuous corticated borders except in the area associated with the roots of teeth 19 through 24. The lesion extends superiorly to include the apical half of the roots of teeth 20 through 22 and the apex of tooth 23, and inferiorly to just above the inferior cortex. The mesiodistal dimension is approximately 2.0 cm, and the superoinferior dimension is 1.5 cm. The lamina dura and periodontal ligament space of teeth 20 through 22 do not appear to be present on this radiograph. Note the configuration of the occlusal plane and the palatoglossal air space. What panoramic technique errors are suggested by this image?

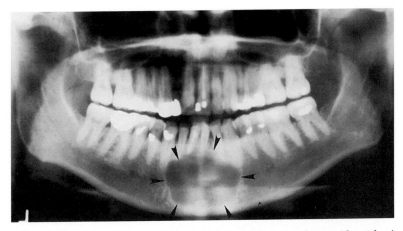

Figure 9–3. A panoramic radiograph demonstrating a single, somewhat ovoid, predominantly radiolucent, unilocular lesion with corticated and slightly scalloped borders *(arrowheads)*. The lesion is symmetrically located across the midline and extends mesiodistally from the apical region of teeth 22 to 27, inferiorly to the inferior cortex, and superiorly to include the apices of teeth 23 through 26. Teeth 23 through 26 appear to have been displaced by the lesion. Tooth 25 shows a root canal filling.

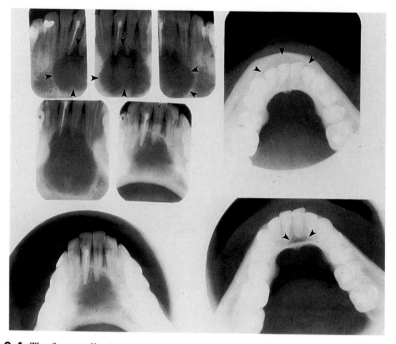

Figure 9–4. The five smaller images are periapical radiographs of the same lesion shown in Figure 9–3. The larger images are occlusal radiographs. Note that the periapical images demonstrate the lesion to have a homogeneous content and a nearly circumferential cortical outline. The PDL space is widened at the apex of teeth 24 and 25, and the lamina dura is indistinct around both apices. The occlusal images suggest that the lesion extends from the buccal to the lingual cortical bone. The upper three periapical images represent the most accurate estimate of lesion size.

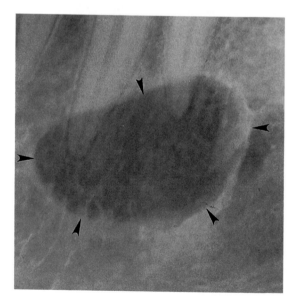

Figure 9–5. A periapical radiograph demonstrating a single, ovoid, unilocular, radiolucent, corticated lesion *(arrowheads)* associated with the root apices of two mandibular single-rooted teeth. The lamina dura and PDL space around both apices appear to be intact and continuous. The trabecular pattern of adjacent bone is visible within the radiolucency. The lesion occupies the middle third of the mandible between the inferior cortex and the alveolar crest and measures approximately 1.5 cm in its mesiodistal dimension.

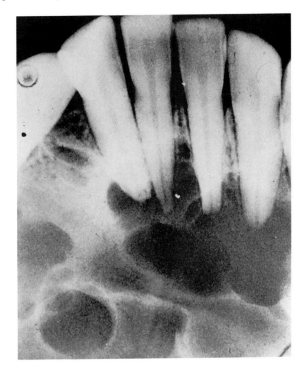

Figure 9-6. A periapical radiograph demonstrating a multilocular, predominantly radiolucent lesion associated with the roots of and causing displacement of teeth 22 through 27. The superior corticated border associated with teeth 23 through 26 extends nearly to the alveolar crest. The lesion extends beyond the coverage provided by this radiograph. A panoramic and/or mandibular occlusal radiograph is/are needed to provide more extensive anatomical coverage.

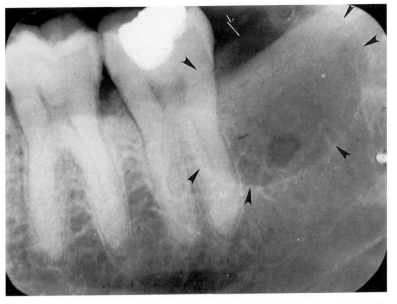

Figure 9-7. A periapical radiograph demonstrating a single, unilocular, predominantly radiolucent, corticated lesion associated with the distal root of a mandibular second molar. The lesion measures approximately 2.0 cm in its mesiodistal and 1.0 cm in its superoinferior dimension. The superior aspect appears to extend above the level of the edentulous ridge in the third molar area. The lamina dura and PDL space of the distal root of the second molar appear unaffected, and the trabecular pattern within the radiolucency appears to be continuous with that of the adjacent bone. A radiolucent zone approximately 0.25 cm in diameter is located inside the lesion's borders. A subtle trabecular pattern is evident inside this more lucent area.

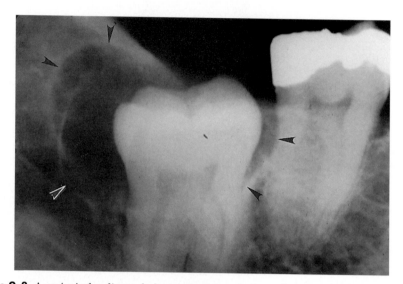

Figure 9–8. A periapical radiograph demonstrating a single, unilocular, corticated, pericoronal radiolucency associated with the crown of what appears to be an unerupted mandibular third molar. The mesial follicular space appears widened to about 2.0 mm, and the distal space has expanded posteriorly approximately 0.5 cm into the ramus. There appears to be no bone overlying the mesial half of the tooth.

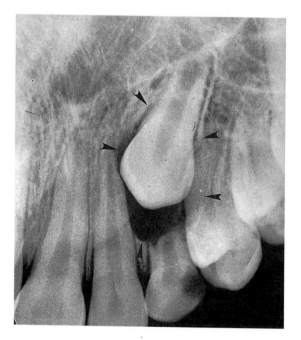

Figure 9–9. A periapical radiograph demonstrating a well-defined pericoronal radiolucency surrounding the crown of an impacted maxillary canine. A cortical outline is not easily visualized. The mesial aspect of the canine has caused displacement of the lateral incisor and resorption of the distal aspect of the lateral incisor root. The radiolucency appears to be 1.5 to 2.0 mm wider than the crown of the canine and extends approximately 4.0 mm toward the alveolar crest. A retained primary canine is present with a large distal carious lesion and approximately half its root remaining.

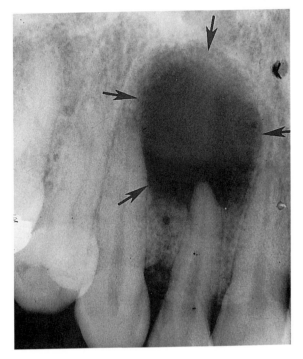

Figure 9-10. A periapical radiograph demonstrating a single, round, noncorticated but well-defined periapical radiolucency associated with the apical third of the root of tooth 7. The radiolucency extends mesially to the distal aspect of the root of tooth 8 and distally to the mesial aspect of the root of tooth 6. The lesion measures approximately 1.0 cm in diameter.

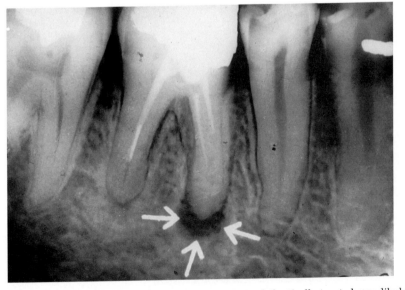

Figure 9-11. A periapical radiograph demonstrating an endodontically treated mandibular first molar. The root canal fillings are significantly short of the apex in each of the roots. A metallic instrument appears to have been fractured and lodged in the distal canal. The periapical area associated with mesial root(s) is affected by a radiolucency *(arrows)* that is continuous with the PDL space. The PDL of the distal root is slightly widened. An area of radiopaque bone (condensing osteitis) surrounds the entire root structure of this tooth.

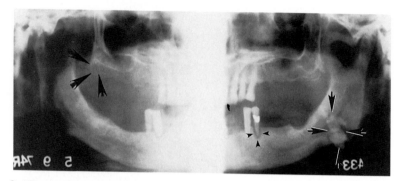

Figure 9–12. A panoramic radiograph of a partially edentulous patient. The arrows on the viewer's left indicate the maxillary tuberosity. The arrowheads at the apex of the mandibular premolar are delineating a well-defined, noncorticated periapical radiolucency surrounding the root. Black and white arrows delineate a mixed radiolucent/radiopaque lesion that is overlying the mandibular canal and inferior cortex just anterior to the gonial angle. The mass measures approximately 2.0 cm superoinferiorly and 1.0 cm mesiodistally.

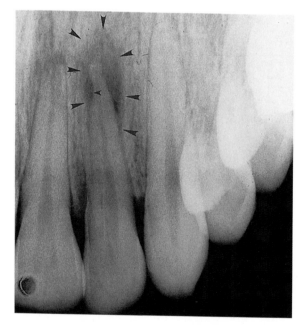

Figure 9–13. A periapical radiograph demonstrating tooth 10 to be affected by a noncorticated, well-defined periapical radiolucency that is continuous with the PDL and encompassing approximately half the length of the root. The mesiodistal dimension is about 0.5 cm and the superoinferior about 1.0 cm. The mesial aspect of the root, approximately 2.0 mm cervical to the apex, has undergone external resorption *(small arrowhead)*, measuring 0.5 mm in depth and 3.0 mm in its cervicoincisal dimension.

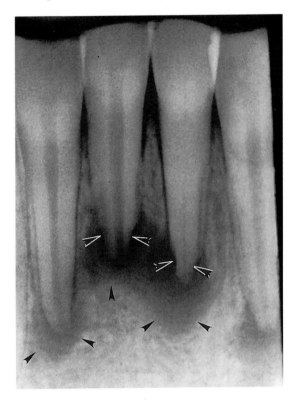

Figure 9–14. A periapical radiograph demonstrating teeth 23 through 26 to be affected by noncorticated, well-defined periapical radiolucencies. The radiolucency associated with teeth 24, 25, and 26 appears to be continuous. Tooth 23 has a separate radiolucency. Black-and-white arrowheads indicate areas of external resorption.

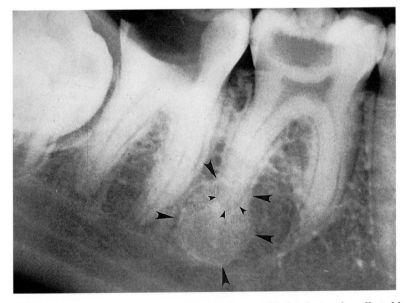

Figure 9–15. A periapical radiograph demonstrating a mandibular first molar affected by a round, periapical radiopacity *(large arrowheads)* at the distal root apex. The radiopacity is approximately 0.75 cm in diameter and exhibits a narrow circumferential radiolucent zone outlined by a cortical border. The contents of the opacity have a uniform granular appearance. The lamina dura and PDL appear continuous and intact around the associated root apex *(small arrowheads)*.

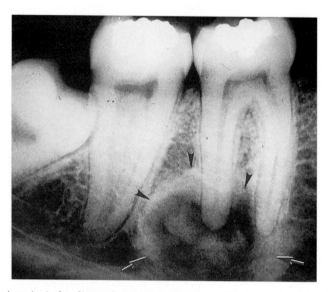

Figure 9–16. A periapical radiograph demonstrating a mandibular first molar with its distal root associated with a mixed radiolucent/radiopaque lesion approximately 1.5 cm in diameter. The borders of the lesion are radiopaque, inside of which is a radiolucent zone surrounding an amorphous radiopaque center. The apex of the mesial root is surrounded by a granular, radiopaque region of bone. The PDL around both roots appears continuous and of uniform width.

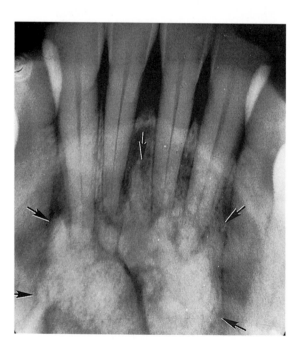

Figure 9–17. A periapical radiograph of the mandibular anterior region demonstrating a mixed radiolucent/radiopaque bone pattern associated with and obscuring the root apices of teeth 23 through 26.

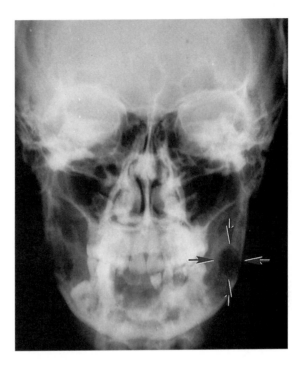

Figure 9–18. A posteroanterior radiograph with a fairly well-defined, circular radiolucency near the mandibular angle, obscuring the inferior alveolar canal in the affected area. The lesion is approximately 1.0 cm in diameter.

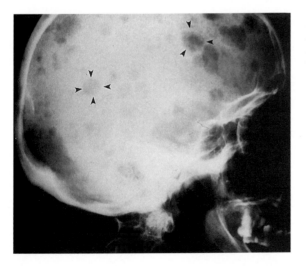

Figure 9–19. A lateral skull radiograph demonstrating several well-defined, or "punched-out," round to ovoid radiolucencies of varying size scattered about the skull.

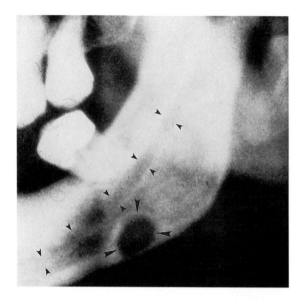

Figure 9–20. A ramus view, lateral jaw radiograph demonstrating a well-defined, corticated radiolucency *(large arrowheads)* located between the mandibular canal *(small arrowheads)* and the inferior cortex in the second molar region. The radiolucency appears to obliterate the inferior cortex.

Figure 9–21. A periapical radiograph of the area of teeth 6, 7, and 8. The alveolar bone level *(arrows)* appears to cross the midpoint of the roots of teeth 7 and 8. Tooth 8 has what appears to be a gutta-percha endodontic filling and an associated, poorly defined, periapical radiolucency *(arrowheads)* that is continuous with the PDL space. The radiolucency contains a radiopaque center.

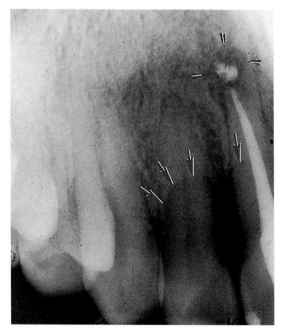

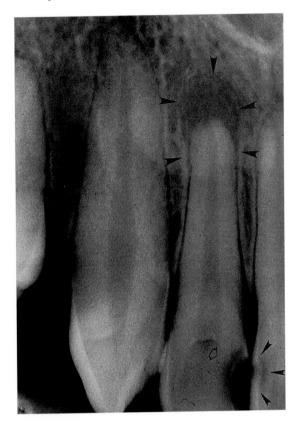

Figure 9–22. A periapical radiograph demonstrating tooth 7 to have a mesial carious lesion encroaching on the pulp *(open arrow)* and a periapical radiolucency *(large arrowheads)* that is continuous with the PDL space. The border around the apical half of the lucency is somewhat indistinct. A faint trabecular pattern is visible within the radiolucency. Tooth 8 exhibits a distal carious lesion *(thin arrowheads)* that extends along the dentinoenamel junction (DEJ) and about halfway to the pulp.

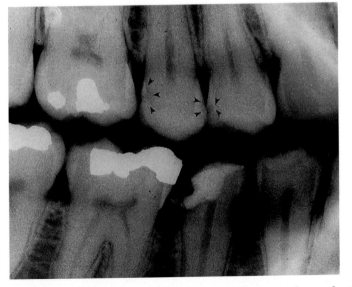

Figure 9–23. A bitewing radiograph demonstrating the maxillary second premolar to have a distal interproximal carious lesion extending approximately halfway to the pulp and an incipient mesial interproximal lesion penetrating less than halfway through the enamel. The first premolar exhibits a distal interproximal carious lesion that extends through enamel and nearly to the dentinoenamel junction.

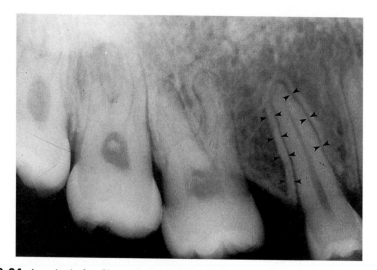

Figure 9–24. A periapical radiograph demonstrating a premolar that exhibits a thickened lamina dura (between the distal row of arrowheads) and a widened PDL space (between the mesial row of arrowheads). Both the lamina dura and PDL space are uniformly affected at the mesial, apical, and distal aspects of the tooth.

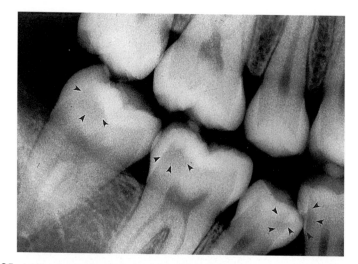

Figure 9–25. A bitewing radiograph demonstrating carious lesions in mandibular molars and premolars. Occlusal caries is approaching the distal pulp horn of the molars. Occlusal caries is approximately halfway to the pulp of the second premolar. Distal interproximal caries, extending slightly more than halfway to the pulp, is visible at the cementoenamel junction (CEJ) of the first premolar, where it is in contact with the mesial marginal ridge of the partially erupted and mesially tipped second premolar.

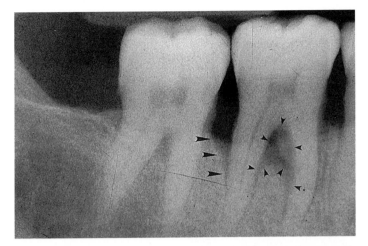

Figure 9–26. A periapical radiograph demonstrating a mandibular first molar affected by a distal vertical bone defect *(large arrowheads)* and bifurcation involvement *(small arrowheads)*.

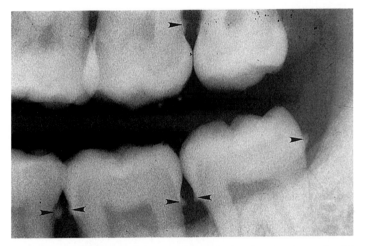

Figure 9–27. A bitewing radiograph demonstrating calculus deposits *(arrowheads)* on the interproximal surfaces of the molars.

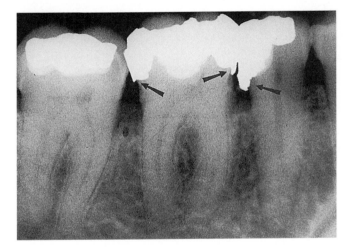

Figure 9–28. A periapical radiograph demonstrating overhangs of interproximal amalgam restorations.

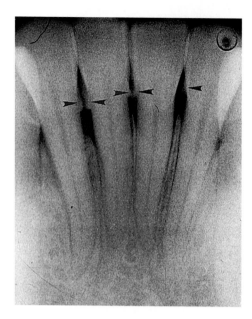

Figure 9–29. A periapical radiograph demonstrating calculus deposits *(arrowheads)* on the interproximal surfaces of the mandibular incisors.

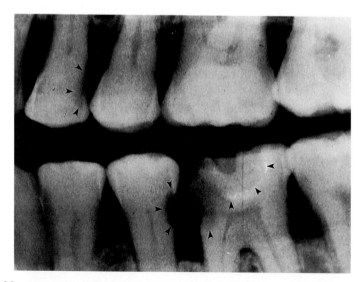

Figure 9–30. A bitewing radiograph demonstrating distal cervical caries *(arrowheads)* of the maxillary first and mandibular second premolars, and occlusal and mesial cervical caries of the mandibular first molar.

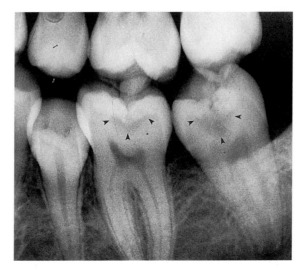

Figure 9–31. A bitewing radiograph demonstrating occlusal caries *(arrowheads)* approaching the pulp of both mandibular molars.

REFERENCES

Coleman GC, Nelson JF: Differential diagnosis of radiographic abnormalities. In Coleman GC: Principles of Oral Diagnosis, p 389. St. Louis, Mosby–Year Book, 1993.

Farman AG, Nortjé CJ, Wood RE: Principles of image interpretation. In Goaz PW, White SC: Oral Radiology: Principles and Interpretation, 3rd edition, p 291. St. Louis, CV Mosby, 1994.

Kasle MJ: An Atlas of Dental Radiographic Anatomy, 4th edition. Philadelphia, WB Saunders, 1994.

INDEX

Note: Page numbers in italics refer to illustrations; page numbers followed by (t) refer to tables.

A

Absolute risk, of cancer, in patient exposed to dental x rays, 87–88
Absorbed radiation dose, 80–81, 82, 83(t)
  in dental imaging, 86(t)
Acetic acid, in fixer solution, 202
Acidifier, in fixer solution, 202
Activator agent, in developer solution, 201
Actual focal spot, on target wafer, at anode end of x-ray tube, 39, *39,* 40, 48
Acute radiation dose, 90
Acute radiation syndrome, 92
Added filtration, of x-ray beam, 35
ALARA dose (as low as reasonably achievable dose), in creation of diagnostic image, 80, 85
Ala-tragus line, patient position relative to, in panoramic radiography, 234(t), *235*
Algorithms, in digital subtraction radiography, 11
  in image-processing encoding operations, 71
  in manipulation of electronic images, 68
Alignment. See also *Alignment and angulation.*
  of x-ray beam, 48
    improper, cone cut artifact due to, 124, 163–164, *164*
    testing of, 48
Alignment and angulation, of x-ray beam, 124
  for bitewing imaging, 145, *146,* 147, *148, 149*
    errors in, results of, *163*
  for occlusal imaging, 148–155, *150–154, 156*
  for periapical imaging, *123,* 124, *128–141,* 144, 144(t)
    errors in, results of, 161, 162, *162, 163*
  improper, results of, 161–164, *161–164*
Allylthiourea, enhancement of sensitivity-speck formation with, 58
Alternating current, 38
  conversion of, to direct current, 38
Aluminum chloride, in fixer solution, 202
Aluminum sulfide, in fixer solution, 202
Ammonium thiosulfate, in fixer solution, 201

Amputation caries, 96, *96*
Analog image(s), 6–7
  conversion of, to digital image(s), 7, *7, 8*
Analog-to-digital converter (frame-grabber), *7, 9, 10*
Analysis operations, in image processing, 71
Anatomical anomalies, dental, intraoral radiography in presence of, 166–168
Anesthetics, topical, as aid to placement of intraoral image receptors, *168,* 169
Angulation, of face of x-ray-tube anode, per Benson line-focus principle, *39,* 40
  of x-ray beam, 124. See also *Alignment and angulation, of x-ray beam.*
    changes in, object localization via, *176, 177*
    errors in, results of, 161–163, *161–163*
Anode, x-ray-tube, *28,* 36, 37
  angulation of face of, per Benson line-focus principle, *39,* 40
  target wafer at, *28, 39*
    focal spot on, *39,* 39–40, 47
      determinations of size of, 48
      image sharpness in relation to, 66
Anomalous dental anatomy, intraoral radiography in presence of, 166–168
Anterior occlusal imaging, mandibular, cross-sectional, *154,* 154–155
  topographical, *153,* 153–154
  maxillary, topographical, 149, *150*
Anterior periapical imaging, 123
Anteroposterior positioning effects, in panoramic radiography, 234(t), *236*
Apron, lead, as protection from radiation, 87, 105, *106,* 107
  storage of, *108*
Arches (dental arches), narrow, intraoral radiography in presence of, 168
Area array detectors, 59
  direct. See *Direct digital radiography (filmless radiography), sensors (receptors) for.*
  fiberoptically coupled, 59
Arm (suspension arm), of dental x-ray machine, 27, *28*
  stability of, testing of, 48
Artifact(s), 155–166, 223–232
  film handling errors and, 160, *160,* 223–226, *224–227*
  film placement errors and, 156, 158–159, *159*

E

O

P

Y